MR IMAGING OF LARYNGEAL CANCER

SERIES IN RADIOLOGY

Volume 23

MR Imaging of Laryngeal Cancer

by

J.A. CASTELIJNS
Department of Radiology

G.B. SNOW
Department of Otolaryngology/Head and Neck Surgery

and

J. VALK
Department of Radiology

Free University Hospital, Amsterdam, The Netherlands

With contributions by

G.J. GERRITSEN
Department of Otolaryngology, Dijkzigt Hospital, Rotterdam, The Netherlands

and

W.N. HANAFEE
Department of Radiodiagnostics, University of California, Los Angeles, USA

SPRINGER SCIENCE+BUSINESS MEDIA, B.V.

Library of Congress Cataloging-in-Publication Data CIP

Castelijns, Jonas A.
MR imaging of laryngeal cancer / by J.A. Castelijns, G.B. Snow, and J. Valk ; with contributions by G.J. Gerritsen and W.N. Hanafee.
p. cm. -- (Series in radiology ; v. 23)
Includes index.
ISBN 978-94-010-5451-5 ISBN 978-94-011-3286-2 (eBook)
DOI 10.1007/978-94-011-3286-2
1. Larynx--Cancer--Magnetic resonance imaging. I. Snow, G.B. II. Valk, J. III. Title. IV. Series: Series in radiology ; 23.
RC280.T5C37 1991
616.99'42207548--dc20 90-27135

ISBN 978-94-010-5451-5

Printed on acid free paper

Table of contents

CHAPTER 2: THE PATTERNS OF GROWTH AND SPREAD OF LARYNGEAL CANCER

CHAPTER 3: THE RADIOLOGICAL EXAMINATION OF THE LARYNX

CHAPTER 4: GENERAL ASPECTS OF MR IMAGING

Foreword

MRI is assuming a dominant role in imaging of the larynx. Its superior soft tissue contrast resolution makes it ideal for differentiating invasion of tumors of the larynx from normal or more sharply circumscribed configuration of most of the benign lesions.

Over ten years ago CT made a major impact on laryngeal examination because it was the first time that Radiologists were beginning to look at submucosal disease. All of the previous examinations duplicated the information that was available to the clinician via direct and in-direct laryngoscopy. With the advent of rigid and flexible endoscopes, clinical examination became sufficiently precise that there was little need to perform studies such as laryngography which merely showed surface anatomy. The status of deep structures by these techniques was implied based on function. Fortunately laryngography is now behind us together with all of the gagging and contrast reactions which we would all like to forget. CT is still an excellent method of examining the larynx but it is unfortunately limited to the axial plane. With presently available CT techniques motion deteriorates any reformatting in sagittal or coronal projections. The latter two planes are extremely helpful in delineating the vertical extent of submucosal spreads. MRI has proven extremely valuable by producing all three basic projections, plus superior soft tissue contrast. Although motion artifacts still degrade the images in some patients, newer pulsing sequences that permit faster scanning are eliminating most of these problems. The details of the larynx are becoming so clear that one can now see the intrinsic musculature of the larynx and identify the causes of any dysfunction.

Dr. Castelijns has analyzed his results covering 44 consecutive patients examined with MRI, 12 of whom had surgery with specimen/MRI correlation. All patients had histological verification of malignancy. The 32 patients who received radiation therapy had extensive clinical examinations which were compared to the radiological imaging studies.

This book will play a vital role in this series in Radiology because it comes from one of the leading institutions of Europe and combines the best of the American and European ideas regarding laryngeal cancer. In Europe, the treatment emphasis is on radiation therapy while in the USA, surgery is usually the treatment of choice.

The authors are from the Netherlands and combine the expertise of Dr. J.A. Castelijns in the Department of Radiology and Dr. J. Valk from the Department of Radiology with the Departments of Head and Neck Surgery, under Dr. G.B. Snow and Dr. G.J. Gerritsen. Dr. Castelijns has a long experience in head and neck imaging and has been interested in larynx for sometime. He performed his thesis in imaging of the larynx. Drs. Snow and Gerritsen bring the imaging information into the clinical arena through their knowledge of surgery. Unfortunately only about a third of their patients received surgery so that some of the correlations are not as precise as one would prefer. On the other hand with the emphasis in Europe being placed on Radiation Therapy the reader is offered a little different view of larynx cancer management than is prevalent in the United States.

In an orderly fashion the reader is taken through laryngeal anatomy, physiology and treatment methods so that when pathology of the larynx is introduced for imaging the reader has a better perspective of meaningful imaging results.

The topic of MR Principals and Radiologic Technique must be kept to a reasonable level or they would occupy the entire book. For those individuals wishing greater detail one might recommend The MRI Manual (Moseby) 1990 by Robert B. Lufkin, M.D. In reality technical advances are being made so rapidly that one can only keep current by attending meetings of the major radiology societies to hear the latest on new pulsing techniques and imaging.

The highlight of the book is in Chapter 7 through 10 which make liberal use of comparisons of CT, MR and whole organ sections of excised specimens. The images are of good quality so that the reader is able to verify the findings described by the authors. In some of the subtle findings the reader can make up their own mind about such controversial things as minimal cartilage invasion. Chapter 10 is a review of radiation therapy in the non-surgical cases and how cartilage invasion is related to occurrences. The follow-up in this group is not as long as one would desire primarily because magnetic resonance imaging of the larynx has not been available for a sufficient period of time. They do, however, point out trends of local recurrence if radiation therapy is used when there is obvious cartilage invasion.

In summary this book fulfils a niche of correlation of the MR imaging with patient management by radiation therapy and to some extent surgery. The effects of the radiologic findings on decision making of the clinician is well covered. By covering all aspects of anatomy, physiology, pathology and treatment about a larynx in a single book, the reader will have a ready reference available for MRI of the larynx.

William N. Hanafee, M.D.
UCLA Medical Center

Introduction

This study concerns the role of magnetic resonance imaging (MRI) in the diagnostic work-up of laryngeal cancer. Our intention in publishing this book is to provide all those physicians involved in the diagnosis and treatment of laryngeal cancer (radiodiagnostician, head and neck surgeon, radiotherapist and oncologist) a detailed study of various aspects of the MR imaging of laryngeal cancer. Radiation therapy and/or surgery are the modalities of choice for the treatment of laryngeal cancer in patients who have not received previous treatment. The choice depends mainly on the risk of tumor recurrence and that of complications, as well as on the functional results after treatment, such as the quality of the voice. The response of laryngeal cancer to radiotherapy is related to general conditions, such as the general physical state of the patient, as well as to local conditions, such as the origin and extent of the tumor, its histological characteristics and the nature of the tissues involved. Tumor infiltration into muscular and in particular into cartilagineous structures increases the risk of therapeutic failures and complications, particularly if high doses of radiation treatment are applied. Surgery, and in particular conservation surgery, requires a detailed knowledge of the superior, inferior and lateral extent of the lesion.

If a choice has been made between radiation therapy and surgery, local properties of the lesion may still influence the plan of treatment. The radiation dose may be adjusted to the TNM staging, anatomic site and volume of the tumor. Reduction of the size of treatment portal forms is an essential part of the planning of the treatment. Similarly, both the procedures of partial and total laryngectomy may be modified according to the extent of the primary tumor within or outside the larynx.

It is evident that accurate assessment of the extent of local disease is of great importance in regard to a correct choice of treatment modality and technique. Laryngoscopic examination reveals a great deal of information of site, volume and extent of the intralaryngeal lesion. However, it does not provide information on the submucosal extension of the lesion and some hidden regions, such as the subglottic area or areas, concealed by a large tumor mass.

Radiological examination can provide additional information on the extent of the disease. The conventional radiological modalities, such as contrast laryngography and conventional tomography, have been largely supplanted by computer tomography (CT). The contribution of CT to diagnostic imaging is based on its ability to visualize much smaller differences in X-ray absorption than conventional radiological techniques and to demonstrate submucosal changes by axial imaging. CT scanning provides useful information about areas that are hidden from visual inspection by bulky tumors, such as the subglottic area. More importantly it reveals submucosal extension which cannot be made visible by other means. It is particularly capable of detecting gross cartilage invasion and of demonstrating extralaryngeal extension.

CT, however, also has its limitations. Its potential to discriminate soft tissues, although superior to that of conventional radiological modalities, still is relatively poor. Furthermore, CT is not adequate to provide an accurate image in the frontal and the saggital planes. CT does not reveal minor cartilage invasion and is incapable of differentiating between post-irradiation fibrosis and recurrent carcinoma.

Of late it has become clear that MRI has the potential to provide additional value in the diagnostic work-up. In condensed phases, liquids and solids, nuclear magnetic resonance (NMR) was first observed by both Bloch and Purcell in 1946 [1,2]. In 1973 MR imaging started to develop, due mainly to the work of Lauterbur, who introduced linear gradients for spatial localisation of NMR signals [3]. MRI is a non-ionizing diagnostic method, providing images with high soft-tissue contrast at any plane of the human body. The density relationships of various tissues are quite different in MRI as compared to CT. CT is based on photon absorption in tissues of different density. MR imaging depends on the presence of hydrogen atoms, certain tissue characteristics and the presence or absence of blood flow.

At the start of our investigations in December 1984, reports on the MR imaging of the larynx were limited to a few examples of normal anatomy of the neck area [4,5]. The techniques of MR imaging of the larynx had certainly not been explored. Comparative investigations between MR images, CT scans and corresponding histopathological sections had not been carried out.

The aim of this study is, first of all, to optimize the MRI technique for the larynx and to describe MR images of the laryngeal anatomy in detail. Subsequently, the potential of MRI to demonstrate the site and extent of laryngeal cancer, and particularly its ability to detect cartilage invasion, is analyzed by comparing MR images with corresponding CT scans and histopathological sections of surgical specimens.

Chapter 1 deals with general aspects of laryngeal cancer. In particular, the therapeutic implications are discussed. Chapter 2 covers the growth and spread of laryngeal cancer, while in Chapter 3 the clinical relevance of various radiological examinations of the larynx, such as conventional tomography, contrast laryngography and computer tomography, are discussed.

Chapter 4 covers the basic principles of magnetic resonance imaging and reviews its technical potentials and limitations. The intent of this Chapter is to provide the practising clinician with a conceptual basis for the underlying principles of magnetic resonance imaging. By design, a certain amount of oversimplification has been used. Chapter 5 goes on to discuss MR imaging techniques of the larynx.

In Chapter 6 we give a detailed description of the axial, frontal and sagittal MR images of normal anatomical laryngeal structures and Chapter 7 deals with MR imaging of laryngeal cancer in previously untreated patients, by comparing pre-operative MRI findings with post-operative histopathological findings in surgical specimens.

Chapter 8 covers a detailed description of MRI of non-ossified and ossified laryngeal cartilages, both normal and invaded by cancer, in untreated patients. Chapter 9 presents an evaluation of MRI and CT results in detecting laryngeal cartilage invasion by cancer in previously untreated patients, by comparing both the CT and MR images with histopathological findings in corresponding sections of surgical specimens and assessing the accuracy of observations performed by CT and MRI observers.

In Chapter 10 the clinical relevance of MRI, especially in regard to findings of cartilage invasion, are discussed in relation to the therapeutical management of laryngeal cancer.

In Chapter 11 our findings regarding the MR imaging of laryngeal cancer are summarized.

References

1. Bloch F, Hansen WW, Packard M. Nuclear induction. Phys rev 1946; 69: 127–131.
2. Purcell EM, Torrey HC, Pound RV. Resonance absorption by nuclear magnetic moments in a solid. Phys rev 1946; 69: 37–42.
3. Lauterbur PC. Image formation by induced local interactions: examples employing NMR. Nature; 242: 191–192.
4. Lufkin RB, Larson SG, Hanafee WN. Work in progress: NMR anatomy of the larynx and the tongue base. Radiology 1983; 148: 173–175.
5. Stark DD, Moss AA, Gamsu G, Clark OH, Gooding GAW, Webb WR. Magnetic resonance imaging of the neck. Normal anatomy. Radiology 1984; 150: 447–454.

Acknowledgments

The authors want to thank Brigitte de Wit, Grace Roquas, Els van der Straten, Lydia Peereboom and Lettie Bergfeld for their secretarial support, and Karin van der Vegt, Adri Mast, Willie Rood, and Ronald Prinsze for their technical assistance in performing the MR examinations.

Chapter 1: General aspects of laryngeal cancer

by J.A. Castelijns, G.B. Snow

1. Introduction

1.1. *Incidence*

Cancer of the larynx is the most commonly occuring malignant tumor in the head and neck area in the western hemisphere. Eighty percent of laryngeal cancers occur in the fifth, sixth, and seventh decades of life; approximately 40% occur in the sixth decade [1, 2].

The general range of incidence rates in the U.S.A. is as follows: glottic, 60 to 70 percent; supraglottic, 25 to 35% and subglottic in about 5%[1, 3]. It is interesting, and as yet unexplained, that the incidence of supraglottic malignant tumors is relatively higher in some other parts of the world; particularly in Finland, Yugoslavia, Italy and the Southeast Asian countries, the 70/30 ratio of glottic to supraglottic involvement is reversed [1, 2].

The incidence of cervical node metastasis with lesions, confined to the glottic region, is very low (about 1%). In contrast, supraglottic and subglottic lesions show a much higher frequency of lymphatic spread: 21–32% [4]. The first nodal stations of lymphatic spread of laryngeal tumors include the jugulodigastric, jugulo-omohyoid and paratracheal nodes [5]. Hematogeneous spread is rare on admission and uncommon. If it occurs, the lungs are the most frequent site of metastatic deposits, followed by the skeletal system [5]. Almost all laryngeal cancers are squamous cell carcinomas (more than 90%) [6].

1.2. *Predisposing factors*

Epidemiological examinations have shown a relationship between excessive tobacco usage and laryngeal cancer. The risk of developing cancer of the larynx has been related to the amount and the type of tobacco consumed. Excessive alcohol consumption in the presence of tobacco use is an additional etiologic factor, particularly in supraglottic cancer [4, 6, 7]. Furthermore, it has been demonstrated that irradiation has a carcinogenic effect [6].

2. TNM staging

2.1. *Introduction*

The two staging systems most frequently used are those proposed by the American Joint Commission (AJC), and by the International Union Against Cancer (IUCC) [5, 8]. Although they differ in several details, these systems are almost identical in respect of laryngeal tumors. The most current and widely accepted classification of carcinoma of the larynx is the TNM staging as proposed by the UICC [8].

2.2. *Clinical classification*

In the classification proposed by the UICC the larynx is divided into three anatomical sites (supraglottis, glottis and subglottis) and these sites are divided into subsites:

A. Supraglottis
  Epilarynx (including the marginal zone)
  (1) Suprahyoid epiglottis
  (2) Aryepiglottic fold
  (3) Arytenoid
  Supraglottis (excluding the epipharynx)
  (4) Infrahyoid epiglottis
  (5) False cords
  (6) Laryngeal ventricles

B. Glottis
  (1) Vocal cords
  (2) Anterior commissure
  (3) Posterior commissure

C. Subglottis

Clinical classification, as proposed by the UICC [8]:

T-staging
Supraglottis:
- T1 Tumor limited to one subsite of supraglottis with normal vocal cord mobility
- T2 Tumor invades more than one subsite of supraglottis or glottis, with normal vocal cord mobility
- T3 Tumor limited to the larynx with vocal cord fixation and/ or invades postcricoid area, medial wall of piriform sinuses or pre-epiglottic tissues
- T4 Tumor invades through thyroid cartilage and/or extends to other tissues beyond the larynx, e.g. to oropharynx, soft tissues of the neck.

Glottis:

T1 Tumor limited to vocal cord(s) (may involve anterior and posterior commisures) with normal mobility
T1a Tumor limited to one vocal cord
T1b Tumor involves both vocal cords
T2 Tumor extends to supraglottis and/or subglottis, and/or with impaired vocal cord mobility
T3 Tumor limited to the larynx with vocal cord fixation
T4 Tumor invades through thyroid cartilage and/or extends to other tissues beyond the larynx, e.g. to oropharynx, soft tissues of the neck.

Subglottis
T1 Tumor limited to the subglottis
T2 Tumor extends to vocal cord(s) with normal or impaired mobility
T3 Tumor limited to the larynx with vocal cord fixation
T4 Tumor invades through cricoid or thyroid cartilage and/or extends to other tissues beyond the larynx, e.g. to oropharynx, soft tissues of the neck.

N-staging
The definitions of the N categories for all head and neck sites except thyroid gland are:
N0 No regional lymph node metastasis
N1 Metastasis in a single ipsilateral lymph node, 3 cm or less in greatest dimension
N2 Metastasis in a single ipsilateral lymph node, more than 3 cm but not more than 6 cm in greatest dimension, or in multiple ipsilateral nodes, none more than 6 cm in greatest dimension, or in bilateral or contralateral lymph nodes, none more than 6 cm in greatest dimension
N3 Metastasis in a lymph node more than 6 cm in greatest dimension

M-staging
The definitions of all M categories for all head and neck sites are:
M0 No distant metastasis
M1 Distant metastasis

The term transglottic carcinoma is used for extensive deep tumor invasion passing the ventricle in vertical direction with subglottic extension. All transglottic carcinomas are characterized by invasion into the paraglottic space [9].

3. Diagnostic aspects

3.1. *History*

Patient's complaints correlate with the intralaryngeal origin of the tumor. Glottic cancers cause hoarseness in an early stage. In contrast, patients with a supraglottic tumor have relatively vague complaints of throat soreness, particularly during swallowing. Sometimes they complain of otalgia ("referred pain") or have noticed a mass in the neck due to lymphatic spread. Patients with a subglottic lesion suffer from vague complaints of coughing in an early stage. In a more advanced stage they may complain of hoarseness, due to infiltration of the vocal muscles or dyspnea due to obstruction of the airway [10].

3.2. *External examination*

Signs of advanced, extralaryngeal tumor spread may be detected by external examination. The assessment of the status of neck nodes is still based on clinical palpation. The fallibility of palpating the neck is well known and large interobserver variations have been reported [11, 12]. The palpability of a lymph node depends on its location, consistency, size, and the type of neck involved. In a neck of average size and in the hands of an experienced examiner, the lower limit of palpability is approximately 0.5 cm in a superficial area such as the submental and submandibular area. Therefore, nodes containing small deposits of carcinoma may not be clinically palpable. Moreover, not all the enlarged lymph nodes contain metastatic deposits [11]. Spread to some regional lymph nodes, such as the paratracheal nodes, almost invariably goes undetected clinically [13].

3.3. *Laryngoscopy*

Indirect and direct laryngoscopic examination reveal a great deal of information about site, volume and extent of the intralaryngeal lesion. Indirect laryngoscopy provides an overall survey of superficial intralaryngeal structures. It does not interfere with the normal mobility, and during phonation the mobility of the cords may be examined. Direct laryngoscopy allows a more precise study of superficial structures. The anterior commissure, the apex of the piriform sinuses and the greater part of the laryngeal ventricles can also be examined. The diagnostic procedure also provides an adequate opportunity for the removal of tissue for histopathological examination. However, laryngoscopy fails to demonstrate the submucosal extent of the tumor. Moreover, some intralaryngeal areas still remain relatively inaccessible, such as the inferior surfaces of the false and true vocal cords and the lateral extent of the laryngeal ventricles [14]. The failure to appreciate the extent of minor subglottic spread is also an accepted limitation of direct laryngoscopy.

4. Therapeutic options

4.1. *Radiotherapeutic options*

4.1.1. Technique

Treatment of patients with laryngeal cancer is performed with megavoltage radiation by left-to-right fields, wedged or unwedged, with the goal of obtaining a homogeneous radiation dose in the target area. The size of the treatment field depends on the T-stage, the extent of the primary tumor, and the presence or probability of the lymphatic spread. The extent of the tumor volume, the degree of differentiation, and the rate of regression of the tumor during irradiation treatment each influence the total radiation dose. The extent of the target volume influences the fractionation schedule.

If lymphatic spread is present, both the primary and the enlarged lymph nodes are treated with a curative radiation dose. Because the supraglottic tumors have a high tendency to metastasize, the first echelon of lymphatic drainage is irradiated electively if invasion is not clinically demonstrated.

4.1.2. *Prognostic factors of irradiation treatment*

The treatment results regarding the locoregional tumor-free survival depends on several factors:

1. The response is related to several general factors, including the physical condition, age, and sex of the patient [15]. Furthermore, the presence of general disease such as diabetes, hypertension, chronic cardiovascular and pulmonary failure and infections in the target volume are risk bearing factors in radiotherapy [16].
2. Other, more local factors, such as location and stage of the tumor and loss of cord mobility influence the response to radiotherapy [17]. Radiotherapy is almost invariably incapable of the sterilization of malignant cells invading the cartilages, other than at the cost of osteomyelitis, chondronecrosis and sequestration of the diseased cartilage [10, 18, 19, 21, 29]. Loss of cord mobility seriously impairs the response to irradiation treatment [19, 22–25].

4.1.3. *Complications due to radiation therapy*

Irradiation treatment of laryngeal cancer may be complicated, sooner or later, by several reactions:

1. In regard to early reactions, it is known that the response of the larynx to radical radiation doses consists of patchy or confluent mucositis, temporary hoarseness and swallowing complaints.
2. Following a larger period of time after the start of irradiation treatment, the cure may be complicated by severe edema and radiation necrosis of bone or cartilages. Complications mainly occur in cases of high fractions of radiation dose, high total dose or due to invasion of bone or cartilage [25, 26].

Furthermore, radiotherapy increases the surgical complication rate of salvage surgery when this has to be carried out to counter recurrent disease.

4.2. *Surgical options*

4.2.1. *Laser therapy and microsurgical stripping*

The carbon dioxide laser provides a precise tool for the excision of endoscopically selected T1 glottic and carcinoma in situ lesions. Whether or not the laser excision is curative depends, amongst other factors, upon the accuracy with which the extent of the disease is estimated. Inadequate exposure, or extension of the carcinoma into the anterior commissure, arytenoid or subglottic area are contra-indications for this approach [27].

4.2.2. *Laryngofissure and cordectomy*
This surgical procedure implies removal of a vocal cord, at times including adjacent subglottic and supraglottic tissue. A malignant T1a-lesion involving the true vocal cord, not extending anteriorly into the anterior commisure and posteriorly beyond the vocal process of the arytenoid cartilage, and having good mobility, can be resected by this method [28].

4.2.3. *Vertical partial laryngectomy*
This implies the removal of nearly all of the ipsilateral thyroid ala with the exception of a vertical posterior strip, together with the vocal cord, ventricle and false cord on one side, but with preservation of the external perichondrium of the resected ala [29]. Usually the anterior commissure is included in the resection. In selected cases this procedure may be extended to include the arytenoid on the involved side or the anterior one third of the contralateral vocal cord.

This procedure is commonly applied in North America as primary treatment for T1 and T2 glottic carcinomas. In most West European countries the application of the procedure is almost exclusively limited to small recurrences of T1 and selected T2 glottic carcinomas after previous radiotherapy [30].

Whatever the indication, the extent of the tumor should fulfill a number of precise criteria. The posterior extension may involve the vocal process or anterior surface of the arytenoid, but it may not involve either the crico-arytenoid joint or the posterior surface of the arythenoid [31]. The tumor may have 8 to 9 mm of subglottic extension in the anterior or midportion of the true cord, but no more than 3 to 4 mm of subglottic extension posteriorly. Extension to the ventricular surface of the false cord indicates a transglottic tumor, which is a contra-indication for partial laryngectomy. Hemilaryngectomy should not be attempted in such cases [32]. All three criteria are recommended, because these findings are often associated with invasion of the thyroid and/or cricoid cartilage: a feature that disqualifies the lesion for hemilaryngectomy because the tumor margins are unpredictable [33, 34].

Some authors report that in selected cases glottic lesions with a fixed cord, fulfilling strict criteria, can be adequately resected by partial vertical laryngectomy [32, 35, 36].

4.2.4. *Antero-frontal laryngectomy for excision of the anterior commissure*
On occasion, the anterior commissure of the larynx will be involved to the extent that radiation therapy is not practical. Such a lesion may be amenable to resection of the anterior commissure. The anterior portions of both vocal

cords and thyroid cartilage, comprising the central segment between two thyrotomies placed about 1 cm on either side of the midline, are excised [23, 37].

4.2.5. *Supraglottic laryngectomy*
Supraglottic lesions, even if they involve the vallecula, base of the tongue, ary-epiglottic folds, and the walls of the piriform sinus, to a level of 1 cm above its apex, should be considered for supraglottic laryngectomy. The lesion should not extend to the lateral pharyngeal wall or into the interarythenoid space. There must be a 5 mm margin between the lower margin of the tumor and the anterior commissure. The true vocal cords and arythenoids should function normally. Invasion of cartilage, other than that of the epiglottis, is a contra-indication for supraglottic partial laryngectomy. It is possible to remove one arytenoid cartilage and fix the vocal cord on this side to the midline, and at the same time preserve laryngeal function [38, 39].

4.2.6. (*Wide-field*) *total laryngectomy*
In the classical technique of total laryngectomy the plane of resection is directly on the laryngeal skeleton. Small tumor masses may be left behind on the deep surface of the infrahyoid strap muscles. It is stated that the wide-field technique of total laryngectomy should be the procedure of choice in all cases. When tumor infiltration is anteriorly extensive, so that the skin appears tethered even the wide-field technique is on its own insufficient. In that case the involved wide skin should be also resected [40].

4.3. *Chemotherapeutic options*

Chemotherapy can be administered to a patient as single agent therapy (methotrexate, bleomycine or cisplatin), combination therapy or combined modality therapy, as an adjuvant to surgery and/or radiotherapy. Chemotherapy has as yet had no significant impact on long term survival and only occasionally offers brief palliation [41, 42]. Integration of chemotherapy into primary treatment of head and neck cancer is still at an investigational stage.

5. Therapeutic management

In various countries, traditional choices of treatment still influence the preferred therapeutic procedures. Whereas in the United States surgery is generally the preferred choice of treatment, in England and Canada irradiation treatment is usually favoured. The reported cure rates vary considerably. The difficulty in staging the primary tumor by laryngoscopy or radiographic methods is likely to be one of the main reasons for this disparity.

T1– and T2–glottic carcinomas

The management of T1 glottic carcinomas is basically decided by the need for optimal conservation of the voice [43]. Vermund has reviewed the results of both surgery and radiotherapy from more than 20 published reports. High cure rates have been reported with either modality. He concluded that glottic T1N0 lesions can be cured very well by adequate radiotherapy with preservation of the voice [44]. Succesful surgical techniques include laryngofissure and cordectomy, partial laryngectomy and CO_2 laser surgery [28, 36].

For T2–glottic lesions, different cure rates are recorded by different institutions [45]. Kirchner reported that cure rates with vertical partial laryngectomy are better than with radiotherapy (71% vs. 35%) [46]. Cocke reviewed reports of 15 major centres, and reported less discrepancy between these modalities (73% vs. 61%) [47].

T1– and T2–subglottic carcinomas

Radiotherapy is preferable in small subglottic tumors [9].

T1– and T2–supraglottic carcinoma

T1–supraglottic and selected supraglottic T2–lesions, which meet the above-mentioned criteria (see 1.4.2.5), are succesfully treated by supraglottic laryngectomy. In general, radiotherapy is the choice of method in the treatment of the other T2 supraglottic lesions [33].

T3– and T4–laryngeal cancer

The recurrence rate after irradiation therapy is much higher with T3 and T4 lesions than with T1 and T2 lesions [20, 44]. Therefore in most centres these advanced tumors are treated with surgery. In most instances this will entail a wide-field laryngectomy, often combined with post-operative radiotherapy [20, 40, 48].

As stated above, partial vertical laryngectomy may be suitable for the occasional fixed-cord lesion that fulfills strict criteria [31–34]. Also, an extended supraglottic laryngectomy has been recommended for selected T3 and T4 supraglottic carcinomas [34].

In contrast, others, like Harwood et al. and Snow et al., hold the view that radiation therapy with surgery in reserve is the preferred treatment for T3 glottic cancer, in view of its potential for laryngeal preservation and better quality of life [10, 18].

Nodal metastasis

Generally, surgery is favoured over radiation therapy for the treatment of regional lymph node metastasis. Because it is preferable to apply the same treatment procedure for both the primary tumor and metastatic lymph nodes, the presence of lymphatic spread will favour the option of surgical treatment [10].

References

1. Bryce DP. Cancer of the larynx. In: Chretien PB, Johns ME, Shedd DP, Strong EW, Ward PH, eds. Head and neck cancer. Saint Louis: The CV Mosby Company 1985:194–195.
2. Ali S, Tiwari R, Snow GB, van der Waal I. Incidence of squamous cell carcinoma of the head and neck. J Laryngol Otol 1986;100:315–327.
3. Ogura JH, Spector GJ. The larynx. In: Nealon TF, ed. Management of the patient with cancer. Philadelphia: WB Saunders Company, 1976:206–238.
4. Ogura JH, Thawley SE. Cysts and tumors of the larynx. In: Paperella MM, Shumrick DA, eds. Otolaryngology. Vol III, Head and Neck. 2nd edition. Saunders Co 1980:2504–2527.
5. Beahrs OH, Myers MH. Manual for staging of cancer. Second edition. Philadelphia: JB Lippincott Company 1983:37–43.
6. Batsakis JG. Neoplasms of the larynx. In: Batsakis JG, ed. Tumours of the head and neck-clinical and pathological considerations. 2nd edition, Williams & Wilkins Co., 1979:135–154.
7. Wynder EL, Bross IDJ, Day E. A study of environmental factors in cancer of the larynx. Cancer 1956;9:86–110.
8. International union against cancer. TNM classification of malignant tumors. Geneva, 3rd edition, 1978, enlarged and revised 1987.
9. Gerritsen GJ. Computed tomography and laryngeal cancer. Academic thesis. Amsterdam: Free University of Amsterdam, 1984.
10. Snow GB, Karin ABMF. Behandeling van larynxcarcinoom. NTvG 1982;126:1096–1100.
11. Ali S, Tiwari RM, Snow GB. False-positive and false-negative neck nodes. Head & Neck Surgery 1985;8:78–82.
12. Sako K, Pradier RN, Marchetta FC, Pickren JW. Fallibility of palpation in the diagnosis of metastases to cervical lymph nodes. Surg Gynaecol Obstet 1964;118:989–990.
13. Bocca E. Conservative neck dissection. Laryngoscope 1975;85:1511–1515.
14. Jafek BW. Fiberoptic endoscopy. In: English GM, ed. Otolaryngology. Revised Edition, Harper & Bow, 1982:572–584.
15. Lederman M. Cancer of the larynx. Part 1: natural history in relation of treatment. Br J Radiother 1971;44:521–525.
16. Bryce DP. Management of laryngeal cancer. J Otolaryngol 1979;8:105–108.
17. Karim ABMF, Kralendonk JH, Yap LY, Njo KH, Tierie AH, Tiwari RM, Snow GB, Gerritsen GJ, Hasman A. Int J Radiot Oncol Biol Phys 1987;13:313–317.
18. Harwood AR. Cancer of the larynx. The Toronto experience. J Otolaryngol 1982;11 (suppl.11).
19. Lederman M. Radiology of cancer of the larynx. J Laryngol Otol 1970;84:867–896.
20. Gerritsen GJ, Valk J, van Velzen DJ, Snow GB. Computed tomography: a mandatory investigational procedure for T-staging of advanced laryngeal cancer. Clin Otolaryngol 1986;11:307–316.
21. Kirchner JA. Invasion of the framework by laryngeal cancer- Surgical and radiological implications. Acta Otolaryngol 1984;97:392–397.

22. Biller HF, Ogura JH, Pratt LL. Hemilaryngectomy for T2 glottic cancers. Arch Otolaryngol 1971;93:238–243.
23. Kirchner JA, Som ML. The anterior commissure technique of partial laryngectomy: clinical and laboratory observations. Laryngoscope 1975;85:1308–1317.
24. Fletcher GH, Jing BS. The head and neck- an atlas of tumor radiology. Chicago: Year book medical 1968:258–265.
25. Harwood AR, DeBoer G. Prognostic factors in T2 glottic cancer. Cancer 1980;45:991–995.
26. Harwood AR, Tierie AH. Radiotherapy of early glottic cancer. Part II. Int Radiot Oncol Biol Phys 1979;5:477–482.
27. Strong MS. Laser excision of carcinoma of the larynx. Laryngoscope 1975;85:1286–1289.
28. Neel HB iii, Devine KD, DeSanto LW. Laryngofissure and cordectomy for early glottic carcinoma: outcome in 181 patients. Otolaryngol Head and Neck Surg 1980;88:79–84.
29. Silver CE. Conservation surgery for glottic carcinoma. In: Silver CE. Surgery for cancer of the larynx 1982:83–121.
30. Croll GA, van den Broek P, Tiwari RM, Manni JJ, Snow GB. Vertical partial laryngectomy for recurrent glottic carcinoma after irradiation. Head & Neck Surgery 1985;7:390–393.
31. Som ML. Cordal cancer with extension to vocal process. Laryngoscope 1975;85:1298–1305.
32. Kirchner J, Som ML. Clinical significance of fixed vocal cord. Laryngoscope 1971;81:1029–1034.
33. Kirchner JA. Two hundred laryngeal cancers: patterns of growth and spread as seen in serial section. Laryngoscope 1977;87:474–482.
34. Hordijk GJ. De behandeling van larynxcarcinoom. Academic thesis, University of Leiden, 1977.
35. Kirchner JA. Treatment of laryngeal cancer. In: Chretien PB, Johns ME, Shedd DP, Strong EW, Ward PH, eds. Head and Neck cancer. Saint Louis: the CV Mosby company, 1985:199–201.
36. Bailey, Stiernberg CM. Surgical management of advanced laryngeal cancer. In: Chretien PB, Johns ME, Shedd DP, Strong EW, Ward PH, eds. Head and Neck cancer. Saint Louis: The CV Mosby company, 1985:207–212.
37. Som ML, Siver CE. The anterior commissure technique. Arch Otolaryngol 1968;87:139–145.
38. Bocca E, Pignataro O, Mosciaro O. Supraglottic surgery of the larynx. Ann Otol 1968;77:1005–1026.
39. Dedo HH. Supraglottic laryngectomy, indications and techniques. Laryngoscope 1968;78:1183–1194.
40. Lam KH. Extralaryngeal spread of cancer of the larynx: a study with whole-organ sections. Head & Neck Surgery 1983;5:410–424.
41. Ross WE. General principles for treatment of cancers in the head and neck: chemotherapy. In: Million RR, Cassini NJ. Management of head and neck cancer- a multidisciplinary approach. Philadelphia: JB Lippincott company 1984;97–105.
42. Snow GB, Vermorken JB, Pinedo HM. Adjuvant chemotherapy: the EORTC trials. In: Bloom HJG, Hanham IWF, Shaw HJ, eds. Head and neck oncology. New York: Raven press 1986:83–92.
43. Karim ABMF, Snow GB, Sick HTH, Njo KH. The quality of voice in patients irradiated for laryngeal carcinoma. Cancer 1983;51:47–49.
44. Vermund H. Role of radiotherapy in cancer of the larynx as related to the TNM system of staging. A review. Cancer 1970;25:485–504.
45. Karim ABMF, Snow GB, Ruys PN, Bosch H. The heterogenity of the T2 glottic carcinoma and its local control probability after radiation therapy. Int J Radiat Oncol Biol Phys 1980;6:1653–1657.
46. Kirchner JA, Owen JR. Five hundred cancers of the larynx and pyriform sinus. Laryngoscope 1977;87:1288–1303.
47. Cocke EW Jr. Management of malignant neoplasms of the larynx. In: English GM, ed. Otolaryngology. Rev ed. vol. 5. Philadelphia: Harper & Row, 1981, Chapter 34.
48. Bardwil JM. Cancer of the vocal cord. Cancer 1972;29:31–36.

Chapter 2: The patterns of growth and spread of laryngeal cancer

by G.J. Gerritsen, G.B. Snow

1. Introduction

Clinical and conventional radiological examination are often insufficient for an exact delineation of the extent of the tumor, particularly in intramural forms without involvement of the mucosa [1]. Histologic examination of large series of surgical specimens after laryngectomy has yielded valuable information on the modes of invasion of laryngeal carcinoma [2–6]. The growth and spread of laryngeal carcinoma are determined by the site of origin of the primary tumor. Local and regional spread is often mechanical in nature. Major factors in determining the direction and extent of the tumor growth are anatomical barriers produced by the laryngeal compartments, the anterior commissure, the cartilagenous framework and intercartilagenous membranes. Within these barriers there are strong and weak points, which may modify the diffusion of cancer.

A topographical classification in which laryngeal carcinomas are divided into three anatomical divisions (supraglottic, glottic and subglottic) is commonly used for a precise description of the extent of the primary tumor. Different modes of invasion will be discussed according to this topographical classification. Furthermore, special attention will be paid to the infiltration in the anterior commissure, cartilage invasion, lymphatic spread and vascular and perineural invasion.

2. Spread of cancer in various regions

2.1. *Cancer of the supraglottic region*

The supraglottic region, according to the UICC-TNM classification rules [7], is bounded inferiorly by the vocal cords and superiorly by the free margin of the epiglottis and by the ary-epiglottic folds. A horizontal line through the lateral angle of the ventricle is considered to be the boundary between the glottic and supraglottic regions (Fig. 1). Most cancers are found on the laryngeal surface of the epiglottis and are localised in the subhyoid portion above the ventricle [8]. The supraglottic cancers tend to be restricted to the supraglottic region. This appears to be related to the embryologic development of the larynx. The supraglottic portion develops from buccopharyngeal anlage, while the glottic and subglottic portions develop from the tracheobronchial anlage [9]. As reported by McGavran and his associates [10],

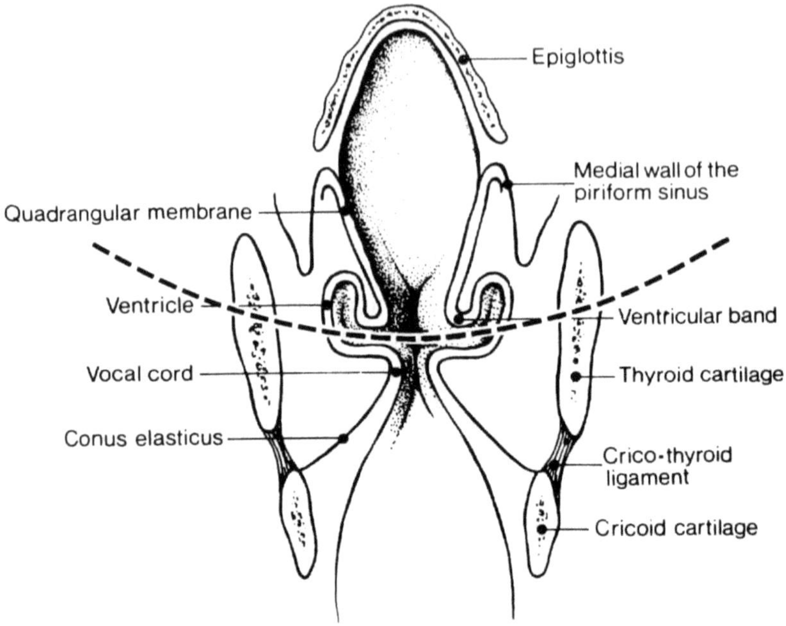

Figure 1. Frontal section of cavity of the larynx.

supraglottic cancers tend to be less invasive than their counterparts in other parts of the larynx. It is generally accepted that supraglottic tumors have pushing margins and only rarely extend to the glottic region [8, 10]. However, spread to the glottic region may occur in carcinomas arising in the ventricle.

The spread of supraglottic cancer, originating at the laryngeal surface of the epiglottis, is superficial and bilateral. Invasion into the pre-epiglottic space (PES) is not uncommon. Tumor spread into the PES cannot be diagnosed reliably by clinical examination, neither is there a reliable conventional radiological technique to demonstrate this growth pattern. Spread into the PES can take place in several ways [4, 5, 11, 12]. Direct passage of the tumor through the orifices of the epiglottic cartilage, destruction of the cartilage or spread through the thyro-epiglottic ligament have been described (Fig. 2). The thyro-hyoid ligament and the hyo-epiglottic ligament are effective barriers against extralaryngeal growth. The spread of carcinomas localised on the ventricular bands is limited. These lesions spread to the laryngeal surface of the epiglottis anteriorly or to the arytenoid posteriorly. Infiltration into the PES is rare, but involvement of the paraglottic space (PGS) is more frequently seen.

Supraglottic tumors do not directly invade the laryngeal framework itself unless the lower edge of the tumor extends to the level of the anterior commissure [4, 6, 8]. However, cancer which invades the PGS can exhibit an agressive growth pattern by infiltrating the laryngeal cartilage and emerg-

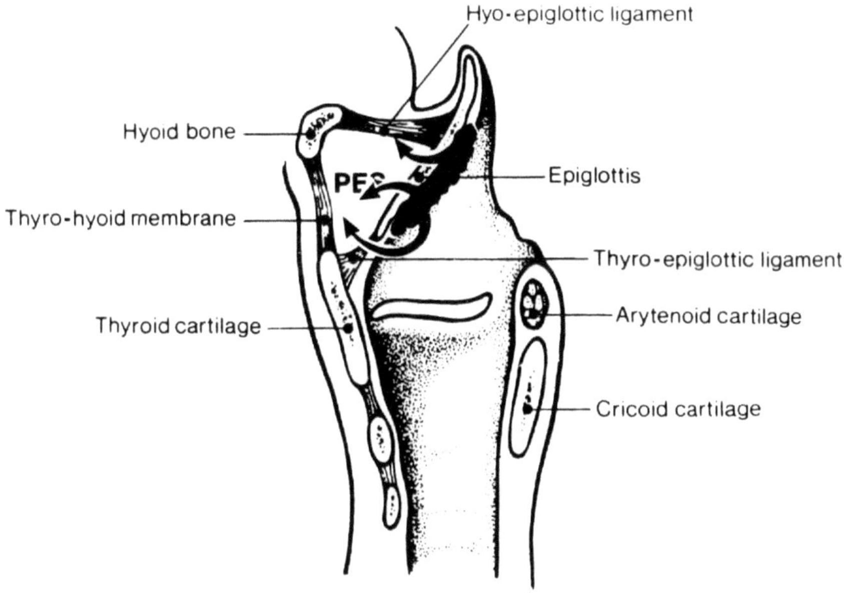

Figure 2. Sagittal section of cavity of the larynx.

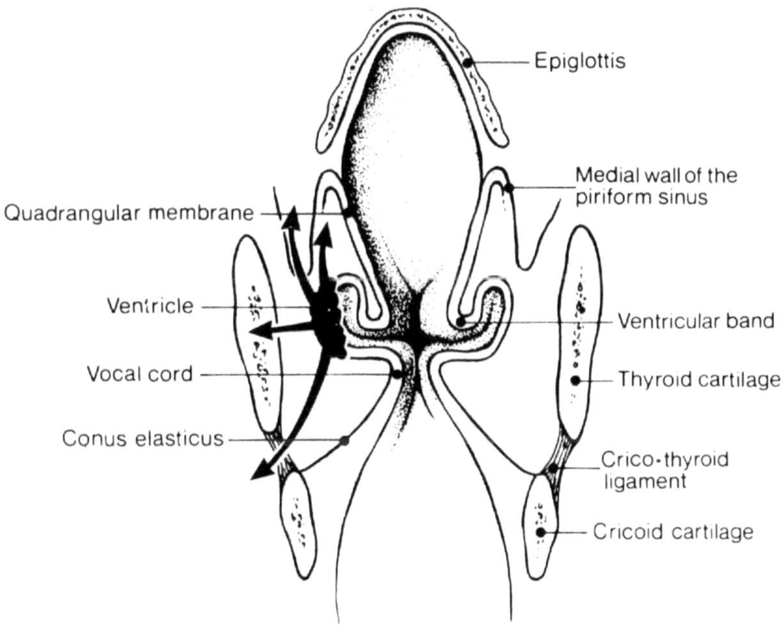

Figure 3. Frontal section of cavity of the larynx.

ing from the confines of the larynx by direct extension between the thyroid and cricoid cartilage or by submucosal spread into the piriform sinus (Fig. 3). The term transglottic carcinoma is used for extensive deep tumor invasion passing the ventricle in a vertical direction with subglottic extension. All transglottic carcinomas are characterized by invasion into the PGS. Spread of supraglottic tumors in a horizontal direction into the PES or in a vertical direction into the PGS is of utmost importance considering the indications for conservation surgical treatment or radiotherapy [13–18]. Precise information on tumor spread must be obtained preoperatively. CT scan can mation on tumor spread must be obtained preoperatively.

2.2. *Cancer of the glottic region*

The glottic region is delineated anteriorly and posteriorly by the anterior and posterior commissure, respectively. The lateral wall of the ventricle represents the superior border and the upper margin of the conus elasticus represents the inferior border (Fig. 4). Most of the glottic carcinomas arise on the free border of the vocal cord which is covered by squamous cell epithelium. There is a predilection for the anterior half of the vocal cords and for the anterior commissure. The posterior commissure, the arytenoid

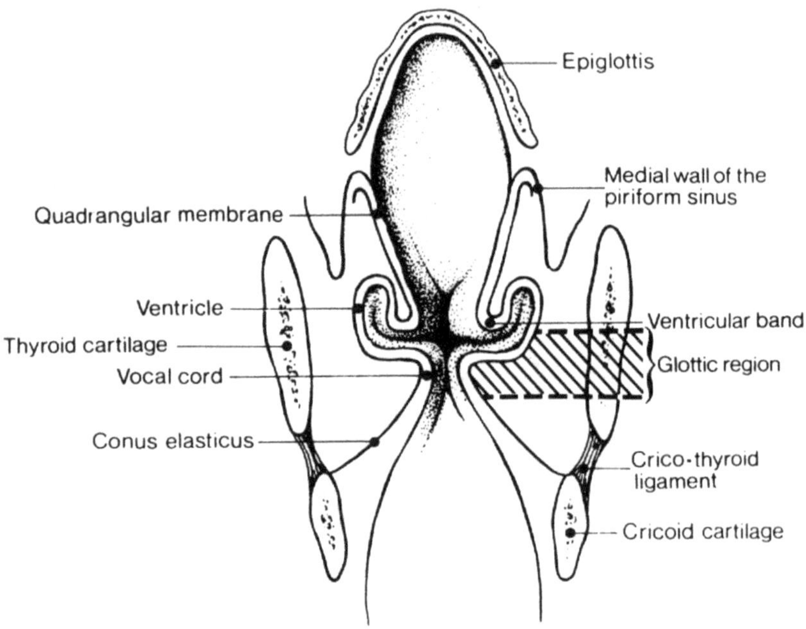

Figure 4. Frontal section of cavity of the larynx.

and its vocal process are rarely primarily involved. However, posterior extension of a vocal cord lesion is possible medially or laterally to the arytenoid cartilages and sometimes results in destruction of the cartilages and the vocal process [4].

The spread of glottic tumors may occur superficially or in depth, in vertical or in horizontal directions. When the spread is superficial the tumor follows the mucosal surface of the free border of the vocal cords. The inferior surface of the vocal cord is frequently involved and submucosal tumor spread into the subglottic region can be present (Fig. 5). The vertical extension of glottic tumors to the supraglottic or subglottic region occurs more frequently than the horizontal extension to the opposite side of the larynx [3, 4, 6].

Vertical extension of the glottic carcinoma to the supraglottic region is frequently related to destruction of the thyro-epiglottic ligament and invasion into the pre-epiglottic space (Fig. 6). Inferior extension into the subglottic region is rarely found below the superior border of the anterior arch of the cricoid cartilage [5]. Subglottic extension in the anterior commissure can result in destruction of the thyro-cricoid ligament and invasion of the prelaryngeal and pretracheal tissues [3–6, 19, 20]. Due to a minor calcification the cricoid cartilage is not frequently infiltrated by tumor [5, 18].

The glottic tumors, if they continue to enlarge, involve the paraglottic space. Extension into the paraglottic space is possible from any mucosa

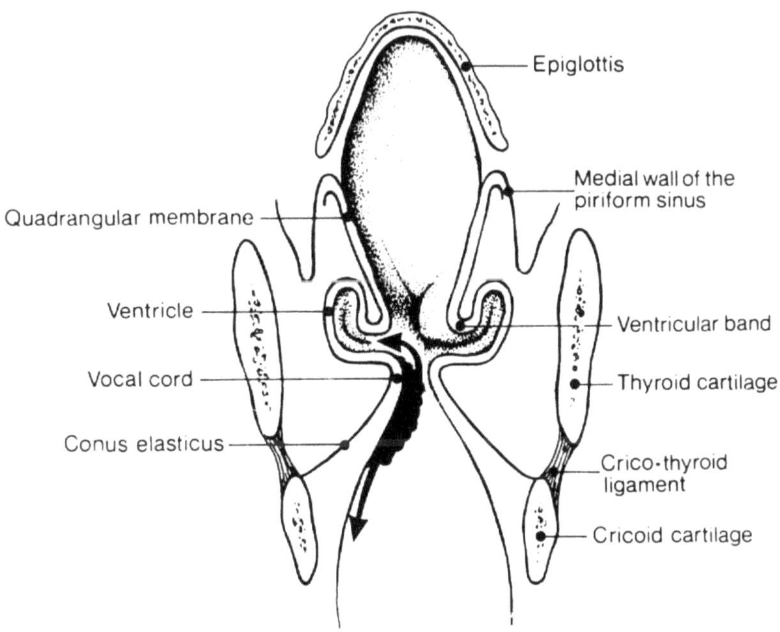

Figure 5. Frontal section of cavity of the larynx.

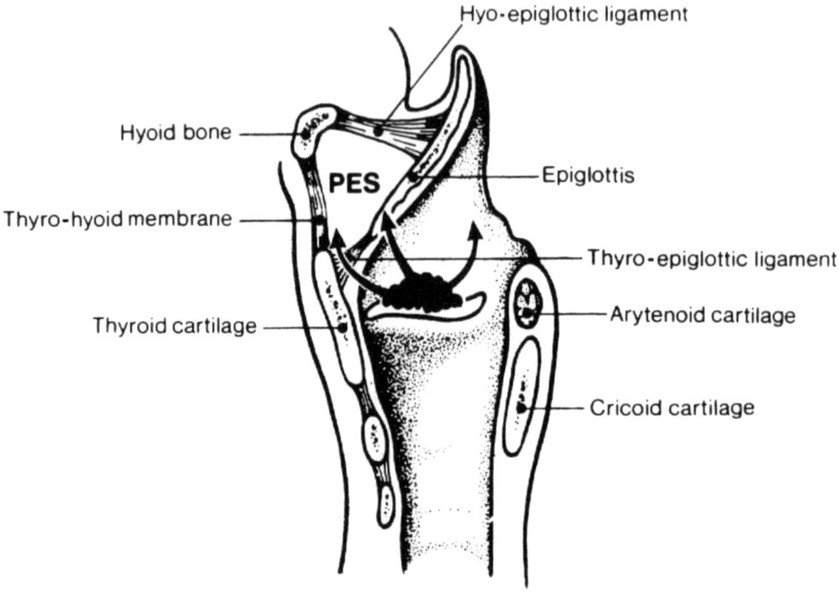

Figure 6. Sagittal section of cavity of the larynx.

adjacent to the PGS. Hypopharyngeal tumors, arising from the medial or anterior wall of the piriform sinus, are also very likely to involve the PGS [5]. Invasion of the PGS means a direct infiltration or destruction of the thyro-arytenoid muscle and the vocal muscle (Fig. 7). Infiltration of the thyroid membrane combined with destruction of the crico-thyroid membrane permits extralaryngeal tumor spread. However, evident cartilage invasion and destruction with breakthrough of the thyroid cartilage and extralaryngeal growth of the tumor is mostly seen close to the midline in the anterior commissure region [21–24] (Fig. 8).

The anterior commissure plays an important role in the spread of glottic carcinomas and therefore deserves special comment. The anterior commissure of the larynx includes the area of the vocal cord insertion at the thyroid alae. The area is delineated superiorly by the upper surface of the vocal cords, and extends 5 mm subglottically. The horizontal boundaries of the area are formed by the thyroid cartilage at the insertion of the anterior commissure tendon and a free margin of 2 mm of the vocal cords in the posterior direction. Since 1942, when Broyles first described the anterior commissure tendon, it has been known that laryngeal carcinoma often breaks through in the anterior midline [25]. There are several reasons for this phenomenon related to the unfavorable anatomical conditions of the anterior commissure region. If the tumor is located in the anterior commissure it is close to the cartilagenous framework. In the anterior commissure there is no

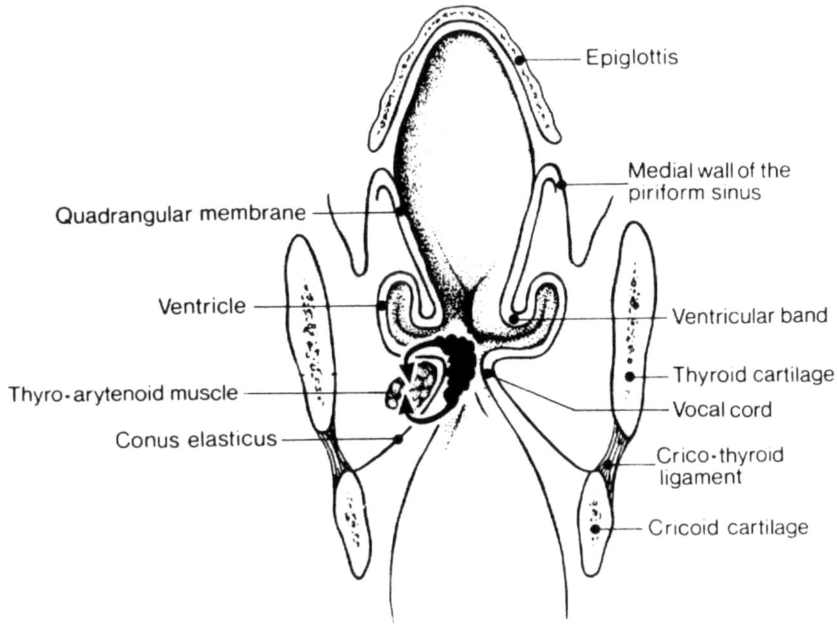

Figure 7. Frontal section of cavity of the larynx.

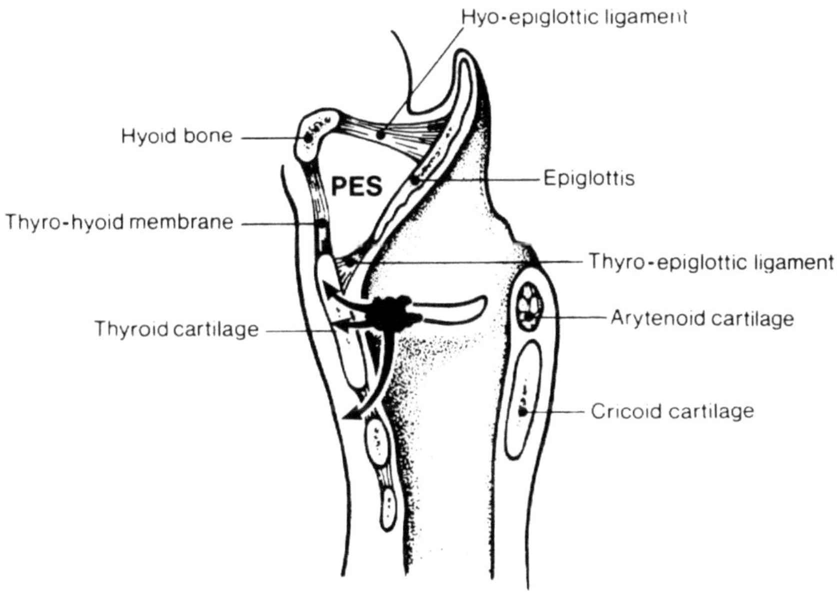

Figure 8. Sagittal section of cavity of the larynx.

protective perichondrial lining inside the thyroid cartilage. In the midline, only a fibrous cord separates the mucosa from the cartilage.

According to Broyles' findings and more recent serial sectioning studies by Olofsson [5, 23], it is clear that the cord or tendon extends from the margin of the thyroid notch down to the level of insertion of the vocal ligament. The perichondrial lining is absent at the insertion of the tendon and tumor infiltration is very likely to occur. However, if tumor spread is confined to the tendon region, metastases to regional lymph nodes are rare, despite the presence of blood vessels and lymphatics. A second weak structure in the anterior commissure region is the crico-thyroid ligament and its insertion at the thyroid cartilage. Destruction of the ligament permits extralaryngeal tumor and lymphatic spread. Evaluation of involvement by tumor of the anterior commissure by conventional X-ray techniques has been proved to be a major problem of this diagnostic method.

2.3. *Cancer of the subglottic region*

The subglottic region is bounded superiorly by the upper margin of the conus elasticus and inferiorly by the lower margin of the cricoid cartilage [26]. The conus elasticus extends from the upper border of the cricoid to the vocal cord where it represents the vocal ligament. Subglottic tumors tend to spread through the conus elasticus into the paraglottic space (Fig. 9). They usually

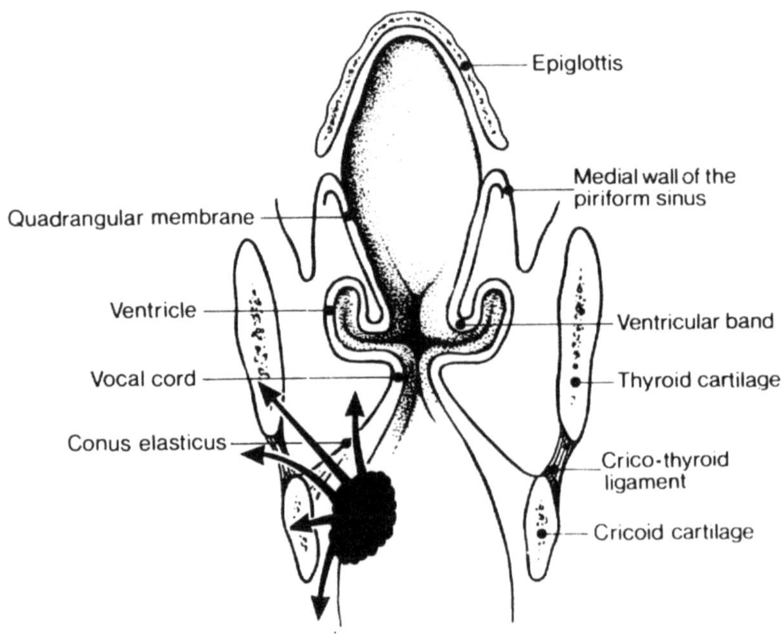

Figure 9. Frontal section of cavity of the larynx.

do not involve the mucosa of the free margin of the vocal cords. Early spread of the disease into the deeper part of the vocal cord will therefore not be detected. Subglottic lesions frequently infiltrate the thyroid and cricoid cartilages. The incidence of invasion, particularly into the thyroid cartilages is 50% or higher [5, 6, 23]. In contrast to supraglottic tumors, subglottic tumors frequently have a submucosal spread with ill-defined outlines. In the posterior direction unsuspected submucosal extension can be found below the level of the cricoid with destruction of the tracheal wall and invasion of the cervical oesophagus. Undetected extension and the tendency to an early extralaryngeal growth, without interfering with cord mobility, provide an explanation for the inaccurate classification of these tumors.

3. Cartilage invasion

Thyroid cartilage invasion occurs most frequently in the lower and middle thirds of the anterior part of the thyroid lamina [6]. Glottic tumors tend to invade the thyroid cartilage in the anterior commissure. As discussed before, the perichondrium is deficient where the anterior commissure tendon attaches the cartilage. Invasion of the cartilages is a well known feature of the transglottic carcinoma.

The mechanism of invasion has been explained by Kirchner [4, 6] and is based on the modes of ossification of the laryngeal cartilages. In most cases, in which cancer invades the cartilage, the invasion is confined to the ossified portions of the cartilage. The ossified areas are better vascularised than the non-ossified portions of the cartilage. The frequency of invasion is related to bone metaplasia, often seen in elderly patients. Infiltration into metaplastic areas evokes a local increase in the number of osteoclasts. These cells destroy the bony patches by resorption in front of the invading tumor. The mechanism is the same as that seen when squamous cell carcinoma invades true bone [27–30]. Infiltration of non-ossified cartilage by tumor is uncommon due to the absence of microvascularisation in the intercellular chondroid substance, the existence of a resistant perichondrial layer and the absence of osteoclasts. Some authors suggest that squamous cell carcinomas provoke osteoclast activity and that local factors are released for the resorption of ossified cartilage [27, 29].

While connective tissue membranes are generally considered as barriers against the spread of laryngeal carcinomas, studies of histopathologic sections have suggested that the same barriers may serve as routes for invasion of the cartilages [31]. This mechanism of invasion will be described. Histologic sections of cartilages in the early stages of invasion show cancer cells growing between collagen bundles of the ligaments and membranes where these are attached to the cartilage [31, 32]. The attachments of the crico-thyroid membrane, the vocal ligament and the anterior commissure tendon are the most common sites. The collagen bundles pass through the entire thickness of the perichondrium and enter the cartilages directly, creating an entrance for tumor invasion. The same mechanism is found at the attachment of the crico-arytenoid joint. The perichondrium itself is a strong barrier to tumor invasion, which is illustrated by the fact that, despite marked lifting or displacement, the perichondrium in most cases is still intact. Large masses of tumor may press against the perichondrium with no evidence of invasion. Detection of cartilage invasion is of great clinical importance. Complications of radiation therapy such as perichondritis, necrosis and subsequent severe edema, are likely to occur when cartilage invasion is present. Demonstration of such an invasion therefore may contribute to better selection of treatment methods.

4. Lymphatic spread

Squamous cell carcinomas of the head and neck in general, and those of the larynx in particular, have a preference for the lymphatic route of metastasis. The incidence of lymph node metastases is dependent on the site of origin and the extent of the primary tumor. The degree of histologic differentiation of the squamous cell carcinoma has also been mentioned as a factor of importance. McGavran has shown that lymphatic metastases are more common when the primary neoplasm is greater than 2 cm. However, the presence of cartilage invasion or invasion into the laryngeal compartments and destruction of membranes and ligaments is not always associated with a higher metastatic rate [10].

Studies by Pressman et al. [3] have demonstrated that the lymph drainage system of the larynx is divided into two compartments according to the embryologic development, which has been discussed before. Some vessels of the superior part pierce the thyro-hyoid membrane and, via the thyro-hyoid plexus, reach the cervical nodes near the bifurcation of the common carotid artery. Others pass through the floor of the piriform sinus, along with the superior laryngeal artery and join the nodes of the chain along the internal jugular vein [33, 34]. Therefore, visualisation of the common carotid artery with its bifurcation and visualisation of the internal jugular vein on CT scan can help to interpret the position, size and number of the adjacent nodes. The vessels of the inferior part form three pedicles. The anterior pedicle pierces the crico-thyroid membrane, drains on the crico-thyroid plexus and passes downwards with the inferior laryngeal artery to the prelaryngeal or Delphian nodes. Some of these reach the supraclavicular nodes where they join the nodes of the chain of the jugular vein. Two posterolateral pedicles pierce the crico-tracheal membrane and drain on the paratracheal nodes and then finally into the superior mediastinum [33–35].

The configuration of the trachea and the related soft tissue structures can be visualised on CT scan [36]. Pathological and normal deep cervical nodes can be scanned. CT scan demonstrates a capacity to show non-palpable enlarged nodes [36–38].

5. Vascular and perineural invasion

Vascular invasion was found less frequently than expected in serial sections by Olofsson et al. [5]. If the tumor is confined to the glottic region no vascular invasion is seen. Vascular invasion can be found in the subglottic extension. The invaded vessels are found immediately beneath the conus elasticus. Vascular invasion of lymph node metastases in the main vessels of the neck can be demonstrated in selected cases. Therefore, preoperative visualisation of lymph node metastases in relation to these vessels is important.

Perineural invasion of laryngeal carcinoma is sometimes found when the lesion infiltrates deeply into the PGS and into the connective tissues deep to the thyro-arytenoid muscle near the lower end of the thyroid ala. In this particular region the branches of the recurrent laryngeal nerve are present.

References

1. Batsakis JG. Neoplasms of the larynx. In: Tumors of the head and neck. Clinical and pathological considerations, Williams & Wilkins Co.,1979. Chapter 9:200–226.
2. Kernan JD. The pathology of carcinoma of the larynx studied in serial sections. Trans Am Acad Ophthalmol Otolaryngol 1950;55:10–16.
3. Pressman JJ, Simon MB, Nonell C. Anatomical studies related to the dissimination of cancer of the larynx. Trans Am Acad Ophthalmol Otolaryngol 1960;64:628–634.
4. Kirchner JA. One hundred laryngeal cancers studied by serial sections. Ann Otol 1969;78:689–693.
5. Olofsson J, van Nostrand AWP. Growth and spread of laryngeal and hypopharyngeal carcinoma with reflections on the effect of preoperative irradiation, 139 cases studied by whole organ sectioning. Acta Otolaryngol 1973;(suppl.308):1–84.
6. Kirchner JA. Two hundred laryngeal cancers: patterns of growth and spread as seen in serial sections. The laryngoscope 1977;87:474–479.
7. International Union against Cancer. TNM classification of malignant tumors. 3rd edition, Geneva, 1978, enlarged and revised 1982.
8. Kirchner JA, Som ML. Clinical and histological observations on supraglottic cancer. Ann Otol Rhinol Laryngol 1971;80:638–644.
9. Tucker GF, Smith HR. A histological demonstration of the development of laryngeal connective tissue compartments. Trans Am Acad Ophthalmol Otloaryngol 1962;66:308–314.
10. McGavran MH, Bauer WC, Ogura JH. The incidence of cervical lymph node metastases from epidermoid carcinoma of the larynx and their relationship to certain characteristics of the primary tumor. Cancer 1961;14:55–62.
11. Ogura JH. Surgical pathology of cancer of the larynx. The Laryngoscope 1955;65:867–871.
12. Bocca E, Pignataro O, Mosciaro O. Supraglottic surgery of the larynx. Ann Otol Rhinol Laryngol 1968;77:1005–1011.

13. Sisson GA, Goldstein JC, Becker GD. Surgery of limited lesions of the larynx. Otolaryngol Clin North Amer 1970;3:529–534.
14. Som ML. Conservation surgery of carcinoma of the supraglottis. J Laryngol Otol 1970;84:655–673.
15. Olofsson J, Williams GT, Bryce DP, Rider WD. Radiotherapy versus conservation surgery in treatment of selected supraglottic carcinomas. Arch Otolaryngol 1972;95:240–248.
16. Kirchner JA. Growth and spread of laryngeal cancer as related to partial laryngectomy. Canad J Otolaryngol 1974;3:460–468.
17. Ogura JH, Sessions DG, Gershon J, Spector MD. Roles and limitations of conservation surgical therapy for laryngeal cancer. Canad J Otolaryngol 1975;4:400–409.
18. Micheau Ch, Luboinski B, Sacho H, Cachin Y. Modes of invasion of cancer of the larynx. Cancer 1976;38:346–353.
19. Szlezak L. Histological serial block examination of 57 cases of laryngeal cancer. Oncologica 1966;20:178–183.
20. Tucker GF. Histological methods for the study of the spread of carcinoma within the larynx. Ann Otol 1961;70:910–916.
21. Kirchner JA. Cancer at the anterior commissure of the larynx. Results with radiotherapy. Arch Otolaryngol 1970;91:524–531.
22. Olofsson J, Williams GT, Rider WD, Bryce DP. Anterior commissure carcinoma. Primary treatment with radiotherapy in 57 patients. Arch Otolaryngol 1972;95:230–237.
23. Olofsson J. Specific features of laryngeal carcinoma involving the anterior commissure and the subglottic region. Canad J Otolaryngol 1975;4:618–623.
24. Bagatella F, Bignardi L. Morphological study of the laryngeal anterior commissure with regard to the spread of cancer. Ann Otol 1971;80:6–13.
25. Broyles EN. The anterior commissure tendon. Ann Otol Rhinol Laryngol 1943;52:342–349.
26. Harrison DFN. The pathology and management of subglottic cancer. Ann Otol 1971;80:6–14.
27. Pittam MR, Carter RL. Framework invasion by laryngeal carcinomas. Head & Neck Surg 1982;4:200–205.
28. Carter RL, Tanner NSB. Local invasion by laryngeal carcinoma. The importance of local (metaplastic) ossification within the laryngeal cartilage. Clin Otolaryngol 1979;4:283–288.
29. Tsao SW, Burman JF, Easty DM, Easty GC, Carter RL. Some mechanisms of local bone destruction by squamous cell carcinomas of the head and neck. Brit J Cancer 1981;43:392–401.
30. Carter RL, Tanner NSB, Clifford P, Shaw HJ. Direct bone invasion in squamous carcinomas of the head and neck. Pathological and clinical implications. Clin Otolaryngol 1980:5:107–113.
31. Yeager VL, Archer CR. Anatomical routes of cancer invasion of laryngeal cartilages. The Laryngoscope 1982;92:449–454.
32. Blitzer A. Mechanisms of spread of laryngeal carcinoma. Bull NY Acad Med 1979;55:813–820.
33. Shaw H. Tumours of the larynx. In: Scott-Brown's Diseases of the Ear, Nose and Throat, 4th edition. Ballantyne J, Groves J. Butterworths, 1979;chapter 15:450–472.
34. Shumrick DA. Neckdissection. In: Otolaryngology. Vol III. Head and Neck, 2nd edition. Shumrick DA, Paparella MM. Saunders Co 1980;chapter 58:2966–2983.
35. Hollingshead WH. Anatomy for surgeons. Vol I. The head and neck, 2nd edition. Harper & Row 1968;Chapter 9:533–541.
36. Mancuso AA, Hanafee WN. Computed tomography of the head and neck. Williams & Wilkins, 1982.
37. Mancuso AA, Maceri D, Hanafee WN. CT of cervical lymph node cancer. Amer J Radiol 1981;136:381–388.
38. Miller EM, Norman D. The role of CT in the evaluation of neck masses. Radiology 1979;133:145–152.

Chapter 3: The radiological examination of the larynx

by J.A. Castelijns

1. Introduction

Radiologists have devised many radiological procedures of varying complexity over a period of many years in order to study the normal and abnormal states of the larynx. These include plain films, tomography, fluoroscopy, cinefluorography, xeroradiography and laryngography [1–5]. In recent years computer tomography (CT) has been added. The following techniques are most commonly used: conventional tomography (planigraphy), contrast laryngography and computer tomography.

2. Phonation manoeuvers

In many radiological techniques for the examination of the larynx physiologic manoeuvers, which will test laryngeal functions, have been used with success. In total, five basic manoeuvers are utilized [1, 6]:

1. Quiet inspiration results in a maximum amount of abduction of the true and false cords;
2. Phonation E. The patient is told to attempt to say "E" softly for a prolonged period of time. The true cords are adducted to the midline, indicating their mobility and configuration. The false cords become paramedian in position. The laryngeal vestibule will open slightly. The piriform sinuses will be in a slightly distended position.
3. Valsalva manoeuver. In this manoeuver the patients are instructed to inhalate deeply and to squeeze with closed lips. The false and true cords come forcefully together in the midline. The subglottic space changes in configuration from an arched roof to a flattened roof. Any disparity between the two sides becomes significant.
4. In the modified Valsalva manoeuver, the patients are instructed to hold their breath and puff out their cheeks. By expiring against pursed lips with a little air being exhaled, the true and false cords are paramedian and the piriform sinuses become distended.
5. Phonation during inspiration or "reverse E". The patient is instructed to make a noise (any noise) while breathing in slowly. The true cords descend and there is lateral distension of the laryngeal ventricles.

3. Frontal tomography

In conventional tomography (or planigraphy) the X-ray tube and the X-ray film are moved in opposite directions so that all points within one specific plane are located in the same position on the film. The structures in this specific plane are sharply defined. The images of the other planes are highly blurred, because the shadows of the structures in these planes are continuously in motion [7]. A frontal tomograph often demonstrates the presence of a lateral subglottic lesion of a vocal cord. Occasionally, minimal subglottic extension may be overlooked or may be indistinguishable from the deformity caused by a bulky tumor of the cord [6, 8]. When the ventricle is well demonstrated, cranial extension of a glottic lesion towards the false cord can be excluded; but when the ventricular air shadow is obliterated, the superior extent of the lesion is often underestimated [8].

In the diagnosis of tumors of the false cords, a frontal tomogram often demonstrates thickening of the false cord, obliteration or depression of the ventricle, and enlargement of the adjacent structures when they are involved. However, it cannot differentiate a tumor mass from edema, as laryngography may do. Frontal tomography has little to offer in the evaluation of the supraglottic lesion originating from the epiglottis.

4. Contrast laryngography

Laryngography is a radiological investigation in which the inner side of the larynx and hypopharynx is coated with a thin layer of contrast medium. With radiographs in antero-posterior frontal and lateral projections during inspiration and phonation, the true and modified Valsalva manoeuvers give good information on endolaryngeal pathology and laryngeal function. A contrast laryngogram can reveal almost all early tumors of the true vocal cords, particularly if the tissues are freely mobile [6, 8, 9]. Thickening and mucosal irregularity of the vocal cord indicate the presence of a tumor. The contrast laryngogram can accurately reveal the presence or absence of subglottic involvement. Any change in the contour of the normal acute subglottic angle indicates the presence of subglottic extension [8]. The ventricle is very well outlined by contrast medium even when it is reduced to a narrow slit [6, 8]. A normal appearance of the false cords between inspiration and phonation manoeuvers and normal distensibility of the ventricle on a reverse phonation manoeuver rule out the possibility of false cord involvement. Fixation of a true cord is well demonstrated by the inspiration and phonation manoeuvers. Contrast laryngography can accurately delineate superficial spread of tumors of the epiglottis or ary-epiglottic folds by showing deformity and distortion of soft tissues and/or mucosal irregularity [8].

However, except for some of the abovementioned blind areas, laryngograms tend to duplicate the information obtained from direct laryngoscopy, particularly with regard to mucosal changes and laryngeal function [6,10]. Furthermore, this diagnostic procedure may cause morbidity due to anesthesia and contrast reactions [8].

5. Computed tomography

The contribution of CT to diagnostic imaging is based on two unique properties:
1. The capability of CT to differentiate much smaller differences in radiological densities than conventional techniques may do;
2. The capability of providing axial images.

CT complements direct laryngoscopy and biopsy better than any other radiological examination. It provides helpful information about areas that may be hidden from visual inspection by bulky tumors, such as the subglottis, the apex of the piriform sinus and the laryngeal ventricle. It reveals deep extension which is not visible by other means. CT helps to clarify suspected pathology in submucosal laryngeal structures, where overlapping structures prevent a full two-dimensional evaluation. Furthermore, it demonstrates nodal metastasis which may not be clinically evident [10, 11]. Caution must be used in diagnosing cartilage invasion by CT because of the random distribution of calcification and ossification within the normal cartilage [12–19]. CT only identifies changes in density, and does not permit a histological diagnosis. Consequently, fibrosis or edema in adjacent tissues can simulate malignant extension on CT [20, 21]. Minor mucosal abnormalities will not be imaged with CT, but this is generally of no clinical importance since such irregularities can be depicted by laryngoscopy. Another shortcoming of CT is its inability to consistently define a transition zone from the true to the false cords. An opened ventricle is not demonstrated by CT in all patients. Spread of the tumor from the false to the true cords, or vice versa, can be difficult to determine on CT [20].

CT fails to demonstrate axial and frontal images in a sufficiently accurate manner. Furthermore, injection of contrast material is needed to detect lymphatic spread. There is also some hazard associated with CT scanning in the form of X-ray exposure and the use of intravenous contrast agents.

6. CT versus conventional radiological techniques

6.1. *CT versus conventional tomography*

Conventional tomography only gives inferential data concerning the submucosal margins of the tumor. CT is superior in showing cartilage invasion and distortions, as well as in showing extralaryngeal extension of the tumor. The diagnostic procedure has largely been supplanted by CT and is regarded as obsolete by some investigators [6, 22, 23].

6.2. *CT versus contrast laryngography*

In a number of different reports it has been stated that CT is more accurate than laryngography in identifying areas of tumor involvement. Deep extension of neoplasms, invading the pre-epiglottic space (PES), paraglottic space (PGS) and the subglottic region can be more directly visualized by CT and do not need to be inferred, as with laryngography [9, 10, 14, 15]. CT provides an additional advantage of direct visualization of laryngeal cartilages [12]. Technological improvements (narrow collimation, rapid scanning time, thinner slices) to CT equipment have provided the means to carry out detailed studies of the larynx during physiological manoeuvers. Functional impairment of the glottis and the arytenoid cartilages can readily be detected by obtaining CT scans during rest, E-phonation, forced inspiration and Valsalva manoeuvers [9, 14, 15, 21].

It has been stated that the laryngeal ventricle is seen in essentially all patients, employing 2 mm thick sections with and without E-phonation [21]. Moreover, CT can compete with laryngography in terms of cost [20]. The patient can be positioned comfortably and no anesthetic is needed. Laryngography will be more reliable in detecting small mucosal exophitic growths. However, the information obtained by laryngography mostly duplicates findings which are obtained by laryngoscopy. It has been concluded by various authors that contrast laryngography is now obsolete [22, 24], or that it should be regarded as an unusual diagnostic procedure [9, 10, 20, 21, 23, 24].

Conventional radiological techniques are available as "fall back" options if necessary. Conventional modalities might still be performed in patients in whom clinical circumstances make it possible to perform direct laryngoscopy under general anesthesia. If a CT scan cannot be performed because of excessive patient motion or unfavourable habitus, one can revert to other diagnostic modalities [23].

References

1. Landman GHM. Laryngografie en cinelaryngografie. De toepassing van contrastmniddelen in de röntgendiagnostiek van de larynx. Academic thesis. Nijmegen: University of Nijmegen, 1966.
2. Doust BD, Tig VM. Xeroradiography of the larynx. Radiology 1974;110:727–730.
3. Fabrikant JI, Dickson RJ. The use of cinefluorography for the radiologic examination of the larynx and hypopharynx in cases of suspected carcinoma. BJR 1965;38:28–38.
4. Pastore RN, May M, Gildersleeve GA. The laryngopharyngogram as a diagnostic aid. Laryngoscope 1964;74:723–737.
5. Woener ME, Braun EJ, Sander I. Xeroradiographic zonography of larynx and hypopharynx. Ann Otol Rhinol Laryngol 1974;83:42–48.

6. Hanafee WN. Radiography of the pharynx and the larynx. In: Valvassori GE, Potter GD, Hanafee WN, Carter BL, Buckingham RA, eds. Radiology of the ear, nose and throat. Stuttgart-New York: Georg Thieme Verlag, 1982: 242–301.
7. Ziedses des plantes BG, Westra D, Penn WM. Methods of examination. In: van Voorthuisen AE, ed. Textbook of radiodiagnosis. Oxford: Oxford University Press. 1979:28–43.
8. Jing BS. Malignant tumors of the larynx. In: Radiol Clin North Amer 1978;16:247–260.
9. Archer CR, Sagel SS, Yeager VL, Martin S, Friedmann WH. Staging of carcinoma of the larynx: comparative accuracy of CT and laryngography. AJR 1981;136:571–575.
10. Mancuso AA, Hanafee WN. A comparative evaluation of computed tomography and laryngography. Radiology 1979;133:131–138.
11. Mancuso AA, Maceri D, Rice D, Hanafee WN. CT of cervical lymph node cancer. AJR 1981;136:381–385.
12. Archer CR, Yeager VL. Evaluation of laryngeal cartilages by computed tomography. J Comput Assist Tomogr 1979;3:604–611.
13. Yeager VL, Lawson C, Archer CR. Ossification of laryngeal cartilages as it relates to computed tomography. Invest Radiol 1982;17:11–19.
14. Gerritsen GJ. Computed tomography and laryngeal cancer. Academics thesis. Amsterdam: Free University of Amsterdam, 1984.
15. Von Zaunbauer W, Haertel M. Zur computertomographischer diagnostik maligner larynxtumoren. Fortschr Geb Rontgenstr Nuklearmed Erganzungsband 1982;136:694–699.
16. Archer CR, Yeager VL, Herbold DR. CT versus histology of laryngeal cancer. Their value in predicting laryngeal cartilage invasion. The Laryngoscope 1983;93:140–147.
17. Hoover LA, Calcaterra ThC, Walter GA, Larsson SG. Preoperative CT scan evaluation of laryngeal carcinoma: correlation with pathologic findings. The Laryngoscope 1984;94:310–315.
18. Silverman PM, Bossen EH, Fisher SR. Carcinoma of the larynx and hypopharynx: computed tomographic-histopathologic correlations. Radiology 1984;151:697–702.
19. Mafee MF, Schild JA, Valvassori GE, Capek V. Computed tomography of the larynx: correlation with anatomic and pathologic studies in cases of laryngeal carcinoma. Radiology 1983;147:123–128.
20. Sagel SS, AufDerHeide JF, Aronberg DJ, Stanley RJ, Archer CR. The Laryngoscope 1981;91:292–300.
21. Scott M, Forsted DH, Rominger CJ, Brennan M. Computed tomographic evaluation of laryngeal neoplasms. Radiology 1981;140:141–144.
22. Ward PH, Hanafee WN, Mancuso AA, Shallit J, Berci G. Evaluation of computerized tomography and laryngography in determining the extent of laryngeal disease. Ann Otol 1979;88:454–462.
23. Mancuso AA, Hanafee WN. Larynx, hypopharynx and cervical nodes- malignant tumors. In: Mancuso AA, Hanafee WN. Computed tomography of the head and neck. Baltimore London: Williams & Wilkins, 1982:26–38.
24. Friedman WH, Archer CR, Yeager VL, Katsantonis GP. CT versus laryngography: a comparison of relative diagnostic value. Otolaryngol Head Neck Surg 1981;89:579–586.

Chapter 4: General aspects of MR imaging

by J.A. Castelijns

1. Introduction

The new diagnostic image modality, magnetic resonance imaging (MRI), has received, and continues to receive, a great deal of attention in the medical community, due to its capability to produce high resolution images with excellent soft tissue contrast in all planes of the human body without the use of ionizing radiation. MRI is based on the principle of nuclear magnetic resonance (NMR). In 1946, Edward M. Purcell and coworkers, of Harvard University, and Felix M. Bloch and coworkers of Stanford University, independently revealed their findings on NMR. The idea of magnetic resonance resulted from the observation that energy is absorbed and subsequently released by nuclei at specific frequencies following excitation by radiofrequency (RF) electromagnetic energy [1, 2]. MRI was developed in 1973, thanks to the work of Paul C. Lauterbur, who published initial experiments on the use of MR to generate an image [3]. Since that time, progress has been very rapid and has enabled the adoption of MR imaging as a standard procedure in medical diagnosis.

2. Technical principles

2.1. *Properties of atomic nuclei*

Magnetism results from the motion of electric charges. Spinning electric charges can produce a magnetic field by their intrinsic spin movement. Protons and neutrons, which compose the atomic nucleus, have an electric charge and a spin motion. Only nuclei having odd numbers of neutrons, protons, or both, have a magnetic moment, because even numbers of nucleons (protons or neutrons) tend to align in such a way that their spins and magnetization cancel. In the case of the spinning proton, the magnetic field can be described as a vector with the direction along the central axis of the spin movement (Fig. 1a).

In the absence of an external magnetic field, the spin axes of many tiny "magnets" are oriented randomly (Fig. 1a). However, if these nuclei are subject to an external magnetic field B0, they will have a tendency to align with the field. Protons (the nuclei of hydrogen atoms) have two possible energy states in the external static magnetic field. The lower energy state is associated with a nuclear magnetic moment pointing along the field (parallel)

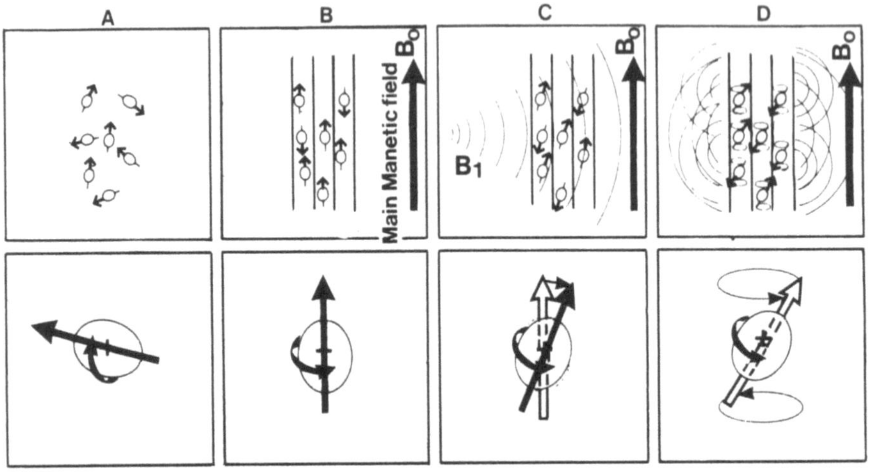

Figure 1. States of proton magnetisation. A. Random; B. Aligned; C. RT-excitation; D. Relaxation. (Courtesy of Luiten et al.)

and the higher one with the antiparallel direction (Fig. 1b). The transition between states involves an exact amount of energy, given a fixed value of the nuclear magnetic moment and a fixed external field strength. The lower energy state is preferred: a slightly greater number of protons have their magnetic moments aligned parallel to the magnetic field (Fig. 1b).

2.2. *Resonance*

Resonance is a property common to all systems that can vibrate. Resonance exists when the excitation frequency coincides with the natural frequency of the system. If the right amount of energy is absorbed or released, transitions between parallel and antiparallel states can occur. The necessary energy can be provided by a magnetic field, because the interaction is with a magnetic field. Such a magnetic field may be obtained by the use of magnetic radiation. The protons can change their orientation if the frequency of the electromagnetic waves and the magnitude of the magnetic field complement each other. If this is not the case, the radiation has little or no effect [4]. When the nuclei, being orientated in the parallel state, are irradiated with electromagnetic energy B0 at the resonance frequency they can take on the antiparallel state (Fig. 1c). They will emit energy, at the same frequency, when they return to the equilibrium (Fig. 1d).

2.3. *Behaviour of a sample of nuclei*

One should in fact consider the magnetic moments of a sample of nuclear spins, rather than that of a single nucleus. The net magnetization vector is zero in the absence of a magnetic field. When the sample is placed into a external magnetic field B0, the nuclei become oriented either parallel or antiparallel to the direction of the applied field. Given the preference for the lower energy state, the net magnetization vector points along the external magnetic field if the field of the main magnet (longitudinal field) is applied to the sample of nuclei. The length of this vector is proportionel to the number of nuclei in the sample and the field strength. Its length and direction characterize the equilibrium magnetization (longitudinal magnetization = Ml) of the sample, i.e. the state that it will eventually revert to after being disturbed. The vector can be disturbed from equilibrium and will align with the net total field by application of a second external orthogonal and superimposed magnetic field B1 (axial field) (Fig. 1c). The net magnetization again returns to the equilibrium state when the superimposed field is removed. The stored energy will be discharged to the environment as radiofrequency (RF) energy (Fig. 1d). The component of the net magnetization, orthogonal to the longitudinal field, is defined as the axial magnetization Ma.

The longitudinal magnetization Ml is reduced from its equilibrium value if the axial field is switched rapidly by irradiation with a resonant frequency emitted by a transmitter coil. The magnitude of the flip angle, e.g. 90 or 180° (a 90° pulse or a 180° pulse) is determined by the duration and intensity of the RF pulse. The longitudinal magnetization has changed into axial magnetization after a 90° pulse (Fig. 2). The magnetization will again return to its equilibrium state in a relaxation process, which can be characterised by tissue parameters: T1 and T2 tissue characteristics. Longitudinal magnetization again increases towards its equilibrium value. This increase is exponential, with a time constant T1 (Fig. 2). One T1 period is that amount of

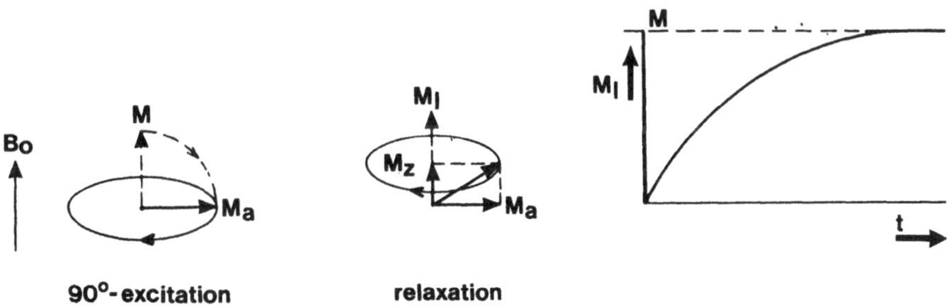

Figure 2. Magnetisation recovery after a 90 degree RF pulse. (Courtesy of Luiten et al.)

time during which 63% of the total magnetization for a particular sample has been achieved, and thus three T1 periods allow almost complete magnetization (95%). During this process transversal magnetization decays exponentionally with a time constant T2. the value of T1 is always longer than T2.

The signal obtained from other nuclei is much less intense than the signal from the hydrogen nucleus. The nucleus which is used for MR imaging is the hydrogen atom, and because the nucleus of the hydrogen atom contains only a single proton the technique of MR imaging may be referred to as proton MR imaging.

2.4. *Proton density, tissue characteristics*

When an RF pulse interacts with protons, its absorption is basically proportional to the proton density. However, rather than differences in proton density, the T1 and T2 tissue characteristics are the primary determinants of relative contrast in MR images. The protons giving rise to an MRI signal are mainly those contained in water and lipid. Protons in large biological macromolecules such as proteins and DNA, and those in solid structures, e.g. bone, have tissue characteristics such that they do not usually contribute to the signal [5, 6]. Fat consists of approximately 50–80% lipid and 10–30% water, whereas the other soft tissues consist of approximately 70–80% water and 5–10% lipid [7]. Medium sized molecules, such as lipids, relax faster than small molecules, such as water, and macromolecules. The relatively widely dispersed H_2O molecules in pure water have a relatively small chance to exchange energy with other molecules in their environment. Efficient relaxation is consistent with short T1 relaxation times. The T1 relaxation time exhibits two extreme values in living tissues: very long T1 times of the order of several seconds in free water, and very short times of approximately 200 ms in lipids and proteins. The relaxation time is indirectly related to the field strength of the main magnetic field. For this reason, when T1 relaxation times are reported, the field strength must be indicated. In contrast, T2 relaxation is less susceptible to the magnitude of the external field. T2 relaxation is more efficient in large molecules. Typically, T2 values in biological tissue have a range from about 50 to 150 ms [8].

Although free water relaxes slowly due to its long relaxation time, the water in biological tissue is found to relax much faster, typically with relaxation times of several hundred milliseconds. A fraction of this water in tissue is bound to the surface of proteins. Rapid equilibrium exists between free and bound water [9]. This equilibrium is probably disturbed in certain pathological conditions. The elevated T1 and T2 tissue characteristics, found in tumors, may be caused by a release of bound water with a concomitant increase of the free water fraction [8, 10].

2.5. *Spin echo technique*

The MR imaging techniques in most common use are the gradient echo and spin echo techniques. The latter is probably the most useful type of MR imaging mode [4]. One of the main reasons for its popularity in MR imaging is that it provides T2 weighted images.

In this technique both T1 and T2 relaxation times contribute to signal intensity and thus to contrast. Several milliseconds (TE/2) after the initial excitation (90° pulse), a second pulse is applied which is strong enough to tip the spins through 180°. The SE sequence can be expressed as (90–T′ – 180–T″ – 90 etc.), at which repetition time (TR) can be defined as T′ + T″ and echo time (TE) as 2 × T′ [4]. Additional echoes can be elicited by applying several 180° pulses in succession.

Manipulation of the equations affords a better comprehension of the dependence of the MRI signal intensity on intrinsic (proton density, T1, T2) and operator-selectable (TE,TR) parameters.

The pixel intensity in MR imaging is a complex function of proton density N(H), T1 and T2 relaxation times, repetition time (TR), echotime (TE) and flow f(v) which can be approximated as follows:

$$I = N(H)f(v)\exp(-TE/T2)(1 - \exp(-TR/T1)).$$

The intensity of the pixel in an MR image is a variable function of four independent parameters.

By proper selection of the programmable sequence parameters, the echo time and the repetition time, respectively, the contrast between suspected pathology and background can be enhanced. From the above equation it can be inferred that the signal intensity increases when

1. T1 decreases
2. T2 increases [8].

It should be more clear, now, given the above, that on MR images the grey scale image contrast between disparate tissues is relative: a tissue may be brighter than its neighbouring tissues due to rapid T1 relaxation or it may be darker because of rapid T2 signal decay. If repetition time is long compared to the longest T1 tissue-relaxation times, then the exp(–TR/T1) term approaches zero. The signal intensity becomes independent of T1 since the magnetization for all protons has completely recovered at the time of the new 90° excitation pulse. The signal is only changed by T2 relaxation processes and possibly by proton density. A repetition time long enough to provide at least three T1 periods is needed. This permits over 95% magnetization. So-called T2 weighted images should have a minimal repetition time of 2000 ms and a minimal echo time of at least 100 ms. If, on the other hand, the echo time (TE) is decreased relative to T2, then exp(– TE/T2) approaches unity. Under these conditions the signal intensity is only dependent on T1. So-called T1 weighted images should have a repetition time equal to the T1 relaxation time (about 500 ms) and an echo time as small as possible [11].

As mentioned above, on images obtained with longer echo times (T2 weighted images vs. T1 weighted images) the MR signal intensity gradually decreases. This diminution of intensity is a manifestation of the signal decrease caused by T2 decay. The relative brightness is usually adapted so as to equalize the overall brightness of the images. The intensity of all tissues diminishes in each subsequent echo; the signals from those tissues with long T2 values decay more slowly than those from tissues with short T2 values. After brightness adaptation, tissues with a long T2 relaxation time will have an increasing absolute intensity in the later echoes, as compared to the intensity in earlier echoes. With increasing echo time the overall signal-to-noise ratio decreases. Therefore images obtained with a longer echo time will have a lower signal-to-noise ratio [8].

3. The equipment

The apparatus consists of several elements that are essential for the production, detection, and display of an MR signal. These include a magnet to produce the static magnetic field, a gradient system, some equipment to produce the varying field, a device to detect the free induction decay (FID) of magnetization, and the electronics to assimilate and display the NMR signal (Fig. 3).

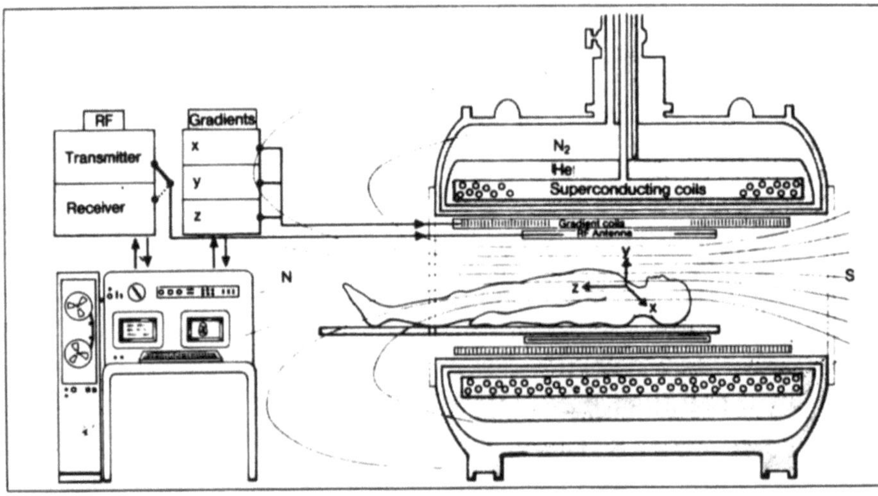

Figure 3. Diagram of generic MR system using a superconductive magnet. (Courtesy of Huk WJ et al., Springer-Verlag, 1990)

A magnetic field is necessary to establish the two "spin" energy states available to hydrogen nuclei. There has been considerable controversy regarding how strong the static magnetic field should be to obtain the best image quality. Although the signal-to-noise ratio for a single excitation increases with field strength, there are several factors that tend to offset this advantage. Firstly, motion artifacts appear worse at higher fields. Secondly, the chemical shift artifact (see next chapter) becomes more striking with increasing magnetic fields.

3.1. *Magnet*

The three major types of magnets are resistive, permanent and superconducting, the last type being the most modern. The superconductive magnets can attain considerably higher field strengths (in the range from 0.35 to 2 Tesla) than resisitive or permanent magnets. The generated field is many thousands of times stronger than the earth's magnetic field, which averages 0.6 mTesla. The wire in the superconductive magnet consists of superconductive material that behaves as a superconductor at very low temperatures and has no significant resistance. The main field of all superconductive magnets is orientated parallel to the long axis of the patient and along the tunnel of the magnet. The superconductive wire and the associated Dewar vessels for the coolant significantly increase the cost of manufacture, service and installation.

3.2. *Gradient system*

A uniform magnetic field and radiofrequency equipment (Section 4.3.3) are needed to perform an MR experiment. However, in order to produce an image, each signal must carry explicit information on its site of origin. This is achieved by manipulating its frequency and phase angle by adding linear magnetic field gradients produced by resistive coils within the imaging volume of the magnet. These linear field gradients are also known as the x, y, and z gradients. The gradient system may be used in association with a selecton of bandwidth and frequency: the z gradient establishes slice thickness and location. During signal collection, the remaining two gradients give x and y coordinates to image pixels [12].

3.3. *Coils*

Resonancy frequency is dependent on the field strength of the magnet. It lies in the frequency range of 5 up to about 85 MHz for various kinds of magnets. A frequency generator capable of generating a varying magnetic field with a wide range of frequencies produces the electromagnetic waves. A frequency (transmitter) coil strengthens and transmits these waves. A second (receiver) coil operates as the receiver for the radio waves emitted by the precessing nuclei. The transmitter and receiver operate through seperate or common antenna coils. Two types of coils are in use in MR imaging: whole-volume coils, which excite and receive signals from a greater part of the body, and local or surface coils, which receive signals from only a small region of tissue. The former type has a much better signal-to-noise ratio.

3.4. *Computer*

The computing system is usually the second most expensive component in an MR system. The production of an MR image depends on a complex cycle of RF excitation and reception and a complex image reconstruction method. MRI requires a flexible and powerful computer for handling the associated tasks of coordination, image computation, evaluation and storage.

4. Disadvantages of MR imaging

4.1. *Claustrophobia*

The long barrel of the magnet induces claustrophobia in about 1–5% of the patients, who consequently refuse to complete the study. Dyspnoeic patients may find the enclosed space inside the imager claustrophobic. Sedation may be a help, but most often gentle persuasion is the best policy. The rejection rate varies from centre to centre, and also varies with the experience of the operators, but can be expected to be less than 2%.

4.2. *Contra-indications*

MR examination is contra-indicated for patients bearing:

1. A pacemaker, which may be affected by the electrical fields generated during imaging, in particular from the gradient fields. The electric field may cause problems in the pacing unit and thus give rise to false pacing signals. This is an obvious and easily avoidable hazard and nobody with a pacemaker should be allowed near the magnet [13]. Another hazard is the force which is exerted on the pacemaker by the static magnetic field. This may cause the patient much discomfort and even harm [14].
2. Aneurysm clips. Any patient with a history of intracranial aneurysm must be carefully examined. Many of the clips used in clipping these aneurysms are ferromagnetic and move in a magnetic field. The risk of detachment

of these clips increases with the magnitude of the static field employed [15].

From experiments with seven different types of widely used metallic stapedectomy prostheses, Applebaum and Valvassori concluded that there is no apparent danger that these prostheses become displaced in stapedectomy patients subjected to the electromagnetic fields of MRI units [16].

It is considered safe to image patients with a history of epilepsy or cardiac arrhythmias.

References

1. Bloch F, Hansen WW, Packard M. Nuclear induction. Phys Rev 1946;69:127–131.
2. Purcell EM, Torrey HC, Pound RV. Resonance absorption by nuclear magnetic moments in a solid. Phys Rev 1946;69:37–42.
3. Lauterbur PC. Image formation by induced local interactions:examples employing NMR. Nature;242:191–192.
4. Valk J, MacLean C, Algra PR. Basic principles of nuclear magnetic resonance imaging. Amsterdam: Elsevier, 1985.
5. Wehrli FW, MacFall JR, Shutts D, Breger R, Herfkens RJ. Mechanisms of contrast in NMR imaging. J Comput Assist Tomogr 1984;8(3):369–380.
6. Young IR, Burl M, Clark GJ, et al. Magnetic resonance properities of hydrogen:imaging the posterior fossa. AJR 1981;137:895–901.
7. Davis PL, Kaufman L, Crooks LE. Tissue characterization. In: Margulis AR, Higgins CB, Kaufman L, Crooks LE, eds. Clinical magnetic resonance imaging. San Francisco, 1983.
8. Wehrli FW, MacFall JR, Glover GH, Grisby N. The dependence of nuclear magnetic resonance (NMR) image contrast on intrinsic and pulse sequence timing parameters. Magnetic Resonance Imaging 1984;2:3–16.
9. Hazelwood CF. A view of the significance and understanding of physical properities of cell-associated water. In: Drost-Hansen W, Clegg J. Cell-associated water. New-York: Academic Press, 1979.
10. Mansfield P, Morris PG. NMR Imaging in biomedicine. New York: Academic Press, 1982:29–30.
11. M. Sprenger. Personal communication.
12. Gademann. Techniques of MR Imaging. In: Huk WJ, Gademann G, Friedmann. MRI of central nervous systems diseases. Berlin: Springer-Verlag, 1990.
13. Pavlicek W, Geisinger M, Castle L, Borkowski GP, Meany TF, Bream BL, Gallagher JH. The effects of NMR on patients with cardiac pacemakers. Radiology 1983;147:149–153.
14. Anonymous. Safety of nuclear magnetic resonance imaging. Lancet 1980;2:103.
15. Finn EJ, Di Chiro G, Brooks RA, Sat S. Ferromagnetic materials in patients: detection before MR imaging. Radiology 1985;156:139–141.
16. Applebaum EL, Valvassori GE. Effects of magnetic resonance imaging fields on stapedectomy protheses. Arch Otolaryngol 1985;820–825.

Chapter 5: MR imaging techniques of the larynx

by J.A. Castelijns

1. Surface coils

Coils which are placed close to the body nearest the organ of interest, so-called surface coils, are a welcome addition in the MR imaging of the laryngeal area [1]. The adjacency of the receiving antenna to the laryngeal area and its small sensitive volume produces a larger signal-to-noise level, at the cost of the magnitude and uniformity of the imaged volume. Such coils enable one to obtain high resolution, thin section images using relatively short acquisition times. With the use of the surface coil it is possible to obtain high resolution images with the minimum technical field of view. A shorter scanning time will reduce motion artifacts due to coughing and swallowing.

1.1. Coil selection

The performance of imaging studies with surface coils remains a challenging task for the radiologist. The best image is produced when the coil spans only the region of anatomic interest. The aim in selecting a coil is to match the region of sensitivity of the coil as closely as possible to the region of anatomic interest [2]. The sensitive region of the coil in the plane parallel to its front is slightly larger than the diameter of the loop. Generally, the sensitivity profile of a surface coil varies in relation to the depth of tissue from the coil surface. Regarding smaller coils the signal-to-noise ratio adjacent to the coil is greater than that of large diameter coils. The depth penetration of a smaller diameter coil is less than that of a coil having a larger diameter coil. Regarding the greater distances from the coil, the signal-to-noise ratio achieved by the larger diameter coils is increased over that of smaller diameter coils. However, only a small improvement in depth sensitivity is obtained by the use of large diameter coils [3]. These principles have a significant impact on the use of coils for the laryngeal area. To image the entire larynx, a coil should be chosen that surrounds the larynx both ventrally and laterally.

Generally the surface coils may have all kinds of configurations, such like half saddle-shaped (Fig. 1), circular, or curved elliptical (Fig. 2). Compared to images made without a coil a significant improvement in signal-to-noise ratio is found on images obtained with a surface coil which is placed in direct contact with the neck region (Fig. 3 versus Fig. 4). However, laryngeal structures (e.g. the cricoid lamina), which are situated more distantly from

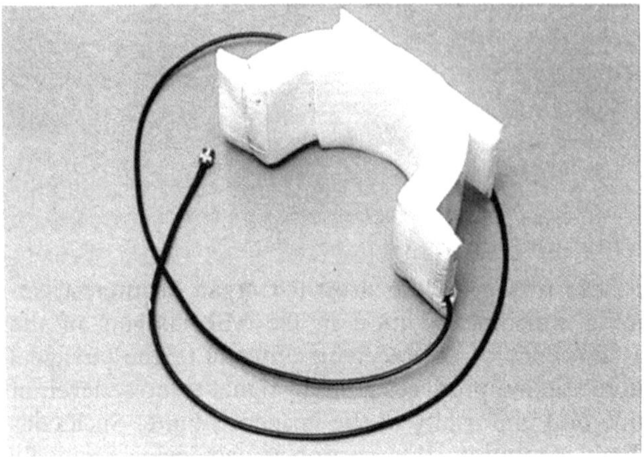

Figure 1. Half saddle-shaped surface coil.

the surface coil, are seen with a lower signal intensity than those adjacent to the surface coil. Furthermore, motion artifacts may frequently occur if the coil has not been immobilized. A half saddle-shaped surface coil (Fig. 5) can surround the anterior and lateral parts of the laryngeal region. The depth penetration of this coil (Fig. 6) is much better as compared with that of the curved elliptical coil (Fig. 4). The half saddle-shaped coil has a better signal-to-noise ratio at greater depths and more uniform brightness. Apart from that, the surface coil can be rigidly mounted and does not contact the patient. This reduces motion artifacts. Positioning problems may become

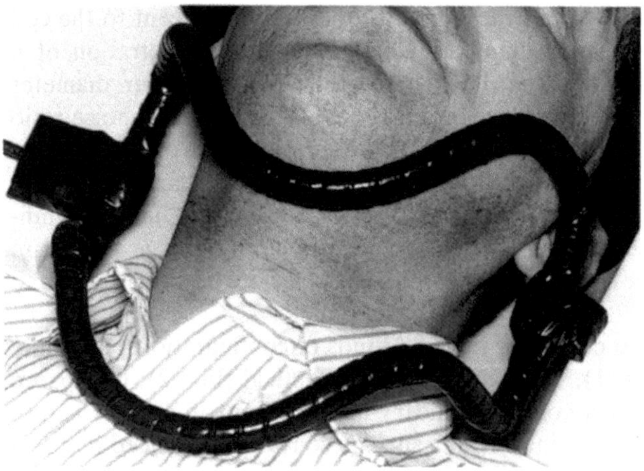

Figure 2. Curved elliptical surface coil.

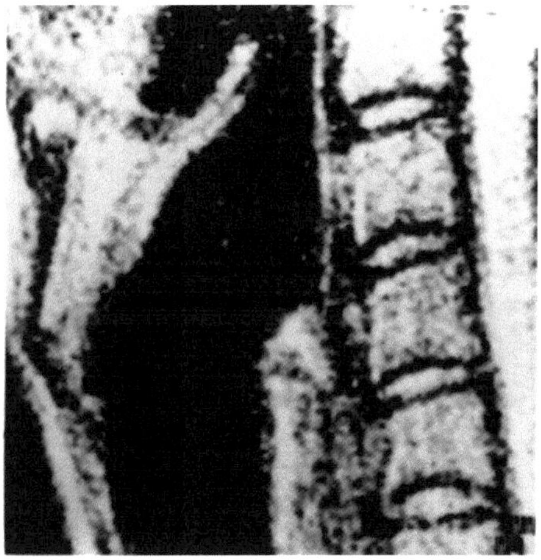

Figure 3. Sagittal image, obtained without a standard head coil.

more severe for smaller, mostly female patients, because the shoulders may hinder adequate low positioning of the coil. Consequently the caudal parts of the larynx are found in the extremities of the region of sensitivity and are imaged with a somewhat lower signal-to-noise ratio.

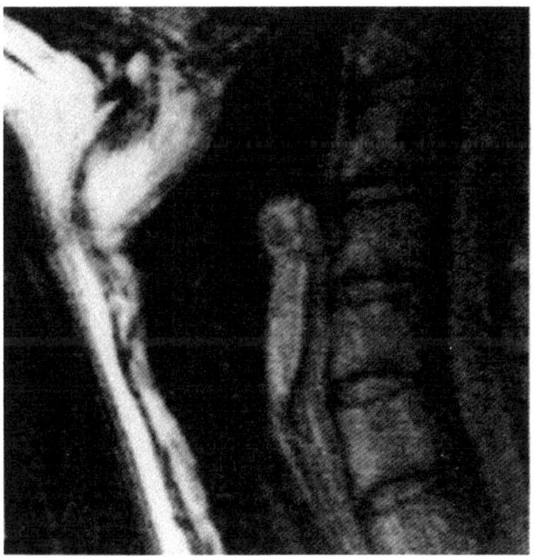

Figure 4. Sagittal image, obtained with a curved elliptical coil.

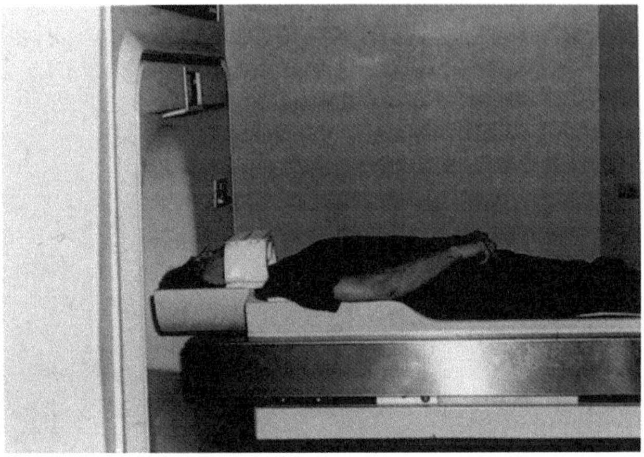

Figure 5. An half saddle-shaped surface coil which surrounds the anterior and lateral parts of the laryngeal region.

2. Parameters

2.1. *Pulse sequences*

The three pulse sequences most frequently used nowadays, which are obtained by combinations of 90 and 180° radiofrequency pulses, are inversion recovery, gradient echo and spin echo. Gradient echo pulses are obtained

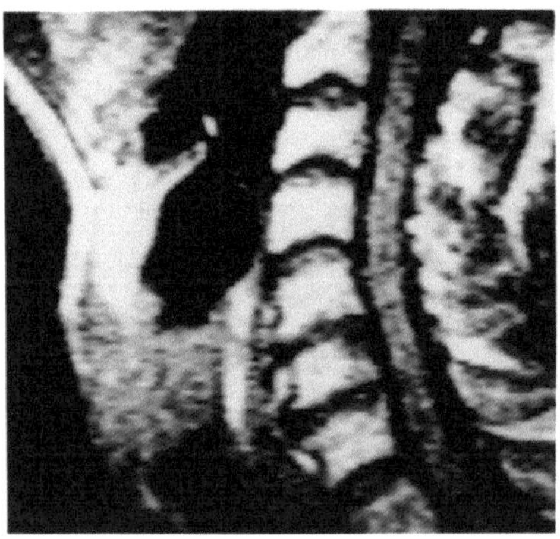

Figure 6. Sagittal image obtained with an half saddle-shaped coil which surrounds the neck anteriorly and laterally.

by tissue stimulation with a lower flip angle (less than 90°). Both gradient echo and inversion recovery techniques are of less value for the laryngeal area.

Soft tissue contrast is better demonstrated on SE images than it is on images obtained by both other MR techniques. Furthermore, the spin echo sequence produces a signal that may depend on both tissue T1 or T2 relaxation time. Tissue T2 values may be among the most sensitive indicators of tissue pathology.

T1 weighted spin echo images (SE 400/32) (TR ms/TE ms) appear to be appropriate to demonstrate laryngeal anatomy and to assess the extent of laryngeal cancer, as will demonstrated in the following chapters. On MR images, accentuating T2 characteristics (proton density or T2 weighted images), tumor is found to have an increased signal intensity in comparison with that found on T1 weighted images. T2 weighted images have a relatively low signal-to-noise ratio. The use of proton density images (SE 1500/32) (TR ms/TE ms) is a good compromise between a reasonable signal-to-noise ratio and an adequate expression of T2 tissue characteristics.

2.2. *Slice thickness*

Several slice thicknesses are available on commercial MR scanners, varying from about 2 to 10 mm. Thinner slices improve the visualization of anatomic detail but require longer scanning times to maintain an equivalent signal-to-noise ratio. Multiple slice acquisition (7 to 9 slices) obtained with 4 mm slice thickness with a 2 mm interslice gap may demonstrate the entire laryngeal region with high anatomic detail of the refined laryngeal anatomy.

2.3. *Slice direction*

An option exist to image in each standard plane or even in oblique planes. The advantage of MR imaging over CT is that the slices may be obtained directly in any of these standard directions without incurring the noisy inaccuracy of reformatting and without moving the patient. The axial imaging technique is, above other scan directions, appropriate to study the site and extent of tumor in the intralaryngeal compartments, the laryngeal cartilages, as well as in extralaryngeal structures, such as the infrahyoid muscles, piriform sinus, subcutaneous fat and lymph nodes along the carotid sheath. Midline sagittal MR images in supraglottic tumors may be helpful to show the proximity of tumor to the anterior commissure and to confirm spread to the tongue base via the anterior commissure. On frontal images the craniocaudal extension is more clearly demonstrated. The laryngeal ventricles may be seen open, but this is not a constant finding in patients who do not have abnormalities at the level of the laryngeal ventricles.

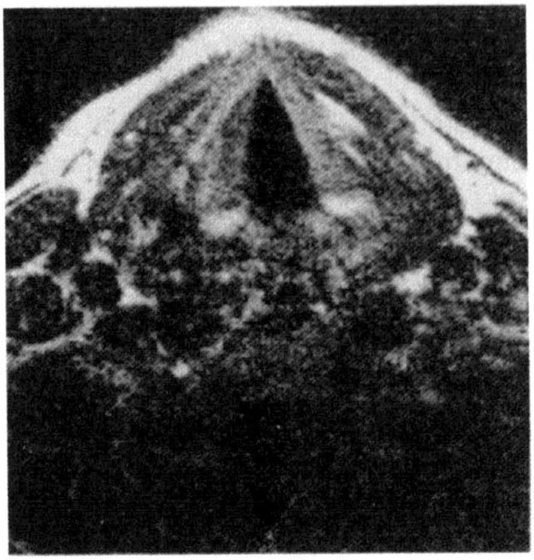

Figure 7. Axial image at the level of the vocal cords, obtained with a 256 × 256 matrix.

2.4. *Matrix size*

Most MR scanners offer various matrices such as 256 × 128 and/or 256 × 192 and/or 256 × 256. Finer matrices improve the visualization of anatomic detail. Scanning time is twice as long for the 256 ×256 than for the 256 × 128 matrices and more signal measurements must be taken to maintain the same signal-to-noise ratio (Fig. 7 vs. Fig. 8). However, images obtained by a

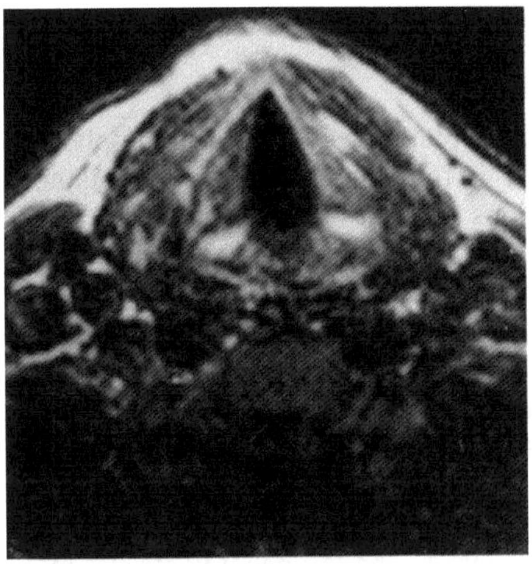

Figure 8. Axial image at the level of the vocal cords, obtained with a 256 × 192 matrix and four measurements.

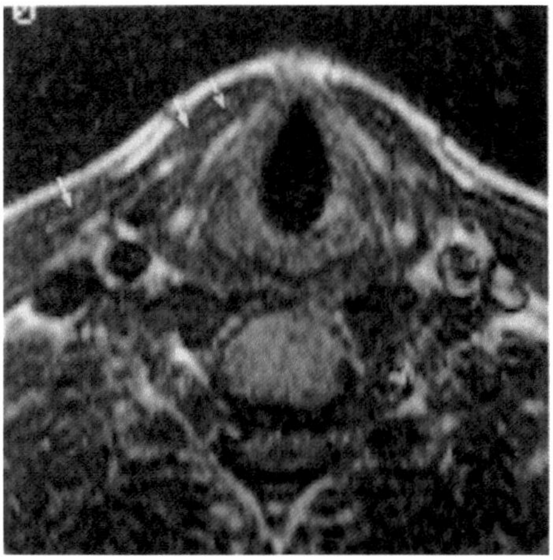

Figure 9. Axial image obtained with a 256 × 128 matrix, which suffers from typical "herringbone" artifacts (arrows).

256 × 128 matrix suffer from typical "herringbone" artifacts (Fig. 9). The selection of an intermediate matrix size (e.g. 256 × 192) may be appropriate in an examination of the larynx. It is important to reduce the field of view as much as possible in order to improve the spatial resolution. A field of view of 180 × 180 mm produces pixels that measure approximately 0.7 × 1.0 mm.

2.5. *Number of signal measurements*

Signal averaging is the best technique to improve MR image quality. The signal is coherent and the total sign will increase with the number of signal averages, also denoted as the number of excitations. On the other hand, noise is, by definition, incoherent and only increases as the square root of the number of scans that are co-added.

At least two and sometimes more signal measurements provide mostly superior images, due to a better signal-to-noise ratio. In a comparison between Figs. 8 and 10 the improvement in image quality due to signal averaging is clearly demonstrated. However, the benefits of signal averaging must be weighed against the increased scanning time required. When many signal averages are taken, scanning time is prolonged and patient movement may erase the gain of more signal measurements.

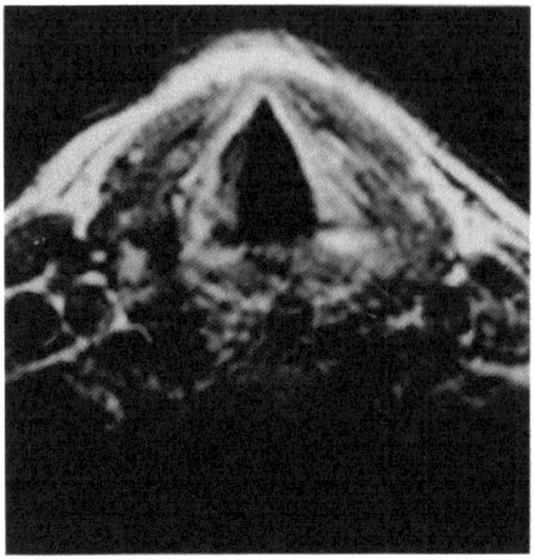

Figure 10. Axial image at the level of the vocal cords, obtained with a 256 × 192 matrix and two measurements.

3. Artifacts

It is important that the interpreter should have some knowledge about the common artifacts encountered in the laryngeal area. A wide variety of artifacts will be discussed. Many are rather obvious. Some artifacts are recognizable as falsifying the image and so misinterpretation can be avoided, but there are several subtle effects that may induce a faulty diagnosis.

3.1. *Motion artifacts*

Motion artifacts are the most common, easily identifiable phenomena that degrade MR images of the laryngeal area. The impact of motion on MR images of the larynx is fundamentally different and substantially more complicated than with CT. Motion artifacts which affect the laryngeal area can be divided into three types:
1. Respiratory motion.
2. Random patient movement (e.g. swallowing, coughing).
3. Fluid motion, due to blood flow in vascular structures.

Motion artifacts due to respiratory movement and to random patient movement may be hard to distinguish from each other.
Both kinds of movement may cause degradation of the image quality. Gross motions (Fig. 11) produce multiple ghosted images. These artifacts usually appear as curvilinear crescents of signal. They outline partial copies of original anatomic interfaces along the phase-encoded direction. An increase in

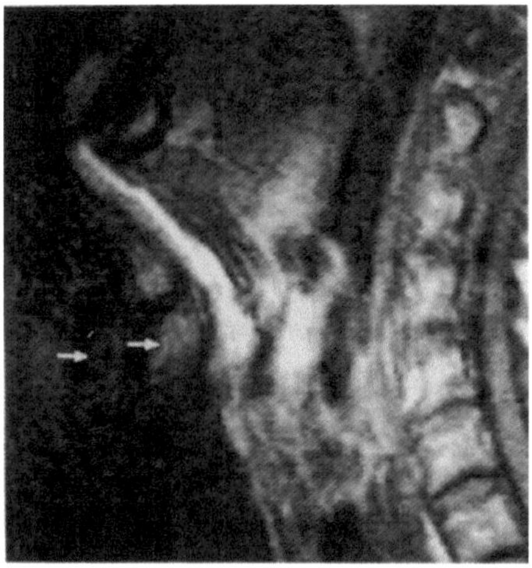

Figure 11. Sagittal image. Gross motions produce multiple ghosted images (arrows).

either the TR value or the frequency of the motion increases the spacing between parent signal and daughter ghosts. More subtle patient motion results in degraded image quality without obvious ghosting (Fig. 12). Motion artifacts are more prominent on images acquired over a long examination time (i.e. a long repetition time). The consequences of the motions differ along the two image axes, the phase- and frequency-encoding axes. Motion ghosts are seen along the phase-encoding axis (normally in the vertical direction of the axial image), irrespective of the direction of the motion. Data

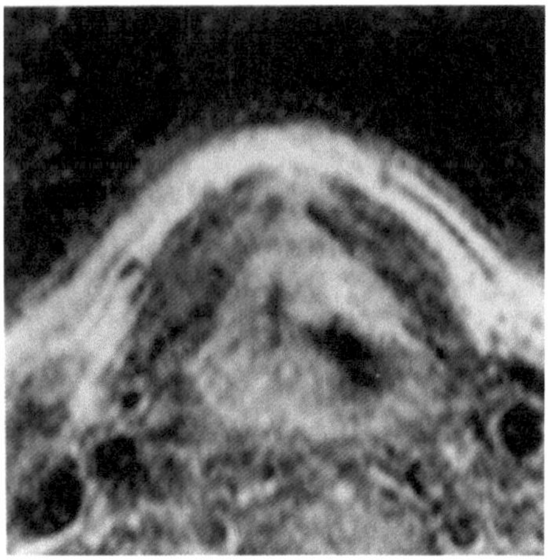

Figure 12. Axial image. Subtle patient motion results in degraded image quality without obvious ghosting.

along the frequency axis (normally in the horizontal axis of the axial image) is obtained in a few milliseconds and motion during this period of time is generally negligible. In contrast, data for the phase-encoding axis spans the entire imaging time. The position and the strengths of the ghosts are determined by the frequency of the motion, not by its amplitude. Certain images in a sequence may be normal and others degraded, if images are obtained by an interleaved slice acquisition mode [4].

Motion artifacts due to respiratory movement may occur if the patient suffers from dyspnea and they do not occur if the patient can breathe quietly. Motion effects can be minimized by short examination times. The use of short examination times necessitates some compromise on image resolution. Explaining to the patient the importance of remaining motionless may reduce the incidence of gross patient movement artifacts. A comfortable gantry and patient positioning, soft lights and sedation may all be used to reduce these artifacts. Motion of the surface coil will induce artifacts. Rigidly mounting the surface coil off the patient eliminates coil motion and improves image quality [4].

Flow artifacts due to fluid motion appear as ghosting in the phase-encoding direction, analoguous to that observed with respiratory motion. The artifacts are shown in a vertical direction. This is a result of signal distortion along the phase-encoded axis, which is in the vertical direction on the axial scan. These artifacts are most prominent for flow occurring perpendicular to the imaging plane. Artifacts due to the flow in the carotid artery results in artifacts as shown in Fig. 13. Because these artifacts mostly stay away from the laryngeal area, they do not interfere with adequate diagnosis of tumor extent of laryngeal cancer [5].

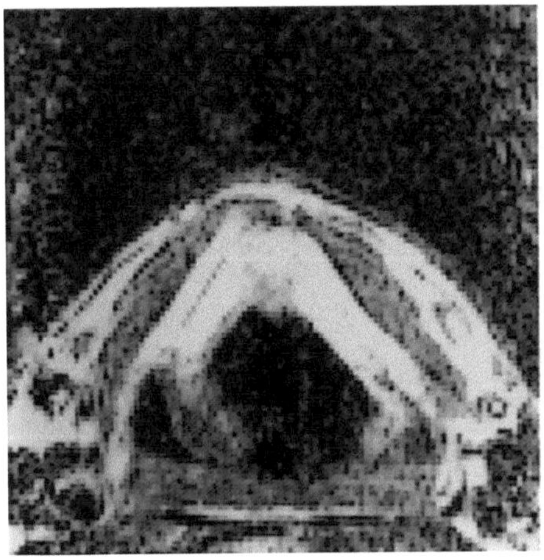

Figure 13. Axial image. Artifacts due to the flow in the carotid artery.

In our experience the use of shorter scanning times allowed MR imaging to provide good diagnostic results in almost all cases. We found an upper limit for a single series of approximately 5–8 minutes, during which time most patients can remain sufficiently immobile. This time limit is constant as the study progresses. In patients with larger lesions, staged as T3 and T4, the presence of movement artifacts interfered in approximately 16% of the examinations in our study group. In patients with smaller lesions adequate diagnosis may be possible in about 90% of the examinations. Strict attention must be paid to patient comfort. One must encourage the patient to remain as immobile as possible. A holder for the coil, which employs a combination of padding for patient's comfort and a mechanical restraint, may also be of some value. By paying more attention to comfort and constraints, it may be possible to perform somewhat longer examinations without image degradation. Although we have not employed sedation or drugs to inhibit coughing and mucous secretion, it may be useful.

3.2. *System artifacts*

Bad machine tuning or field inhomogenities may induce system artifacts. Improper tuning of the RF coil with respect to the laryngeal area may result in a noisy image. If the edges of the laryngeal area are situated at the edge of the coil, a similar effect may be seen at the extremes of the part being scanned (e.g., the first and last slice). On a sagittal image the area around the coil wire is seen as an artifact with a local absence and a decrease of signal intensity in this area (Fig. 14). These areas of signal void or lines of

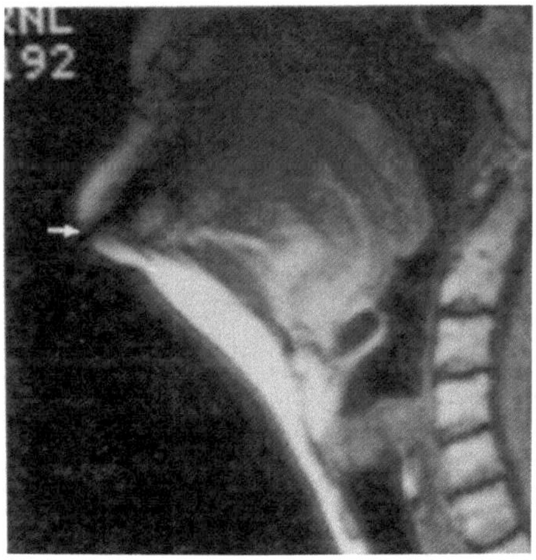

Figure 14. A sagittal image. The area (arrow) around the coil wire is seen as an artifact with a local absence and decrease of signal intensity in this area.

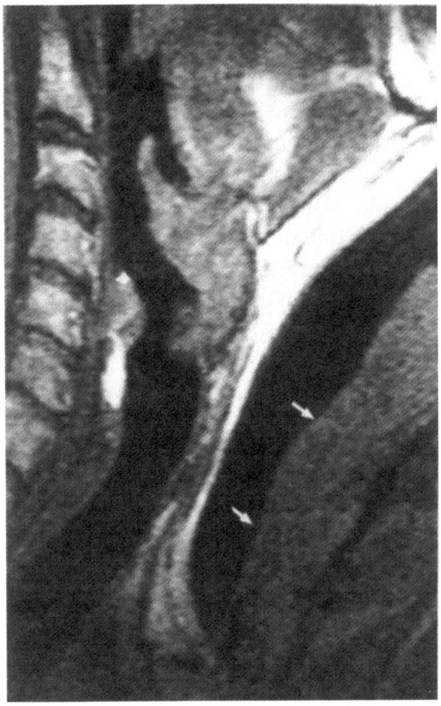

Figure 15. Sagittal image. Wrap-around artifact (arrows).

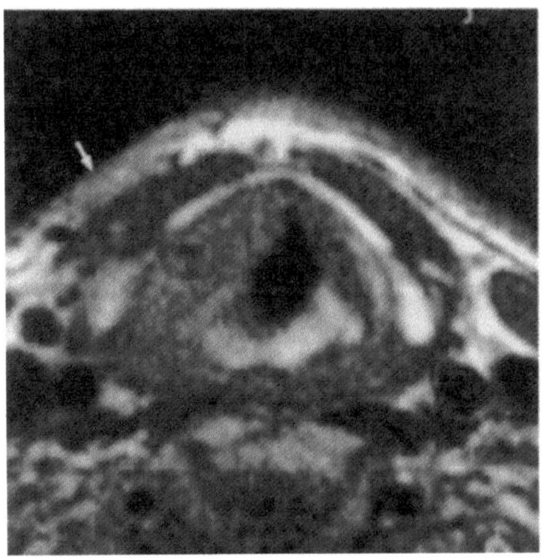

Figure 16. Axial image. Focal change in signal intensity of fat (arrow) due to inhomogenities in the RF field.

null sensitivity are seen when the field of view exceeds the coil dimensions. Touching of the surface coil to a part of the body induces impedance mismatch and mistuning of the coil. This results in a noisy, distorted image [5].

The problem of image "wrap-around" occurs when the region of sensitivity of the coil is larger than the field of view; that portion of the object outside the field of view will be wrapped around or redisplayed onto the opposite side of the cross-sectional image (Fig. 15). This effect is technically referred to as aliasing. It may prove possible, however, to minimize this problem by choosing the direction of the frequency-encoding gradient to coincide with the greater dimension of the coil's region of interest or of the object itself [6]. Generally this artifact does not interfere with adequate diagnosis of the laryngeal area.

Inhomogenities in the RF field may cause protons to be "flipped" by different amounts for the same pulse. This may result in focal changes in signal intensity (Fig. 16). These kinds of artifacts may cause diagnostic problems, especially if they concern focal changes in signal intensity of fat. As will be explained in the following chapters, tumor invading bone marrow will be shown on T1 weighted images with an intermediate signal intensity. However, in case of focal changes of fat, subcutaneous fat may be involved in a manner which is not typical of tumor spread [4].

3.3. *Chemical shift artifacts*

This effect arises when nuclei in different chemical environments have different Larmor frequencies. A very slight but significant difference in resonant

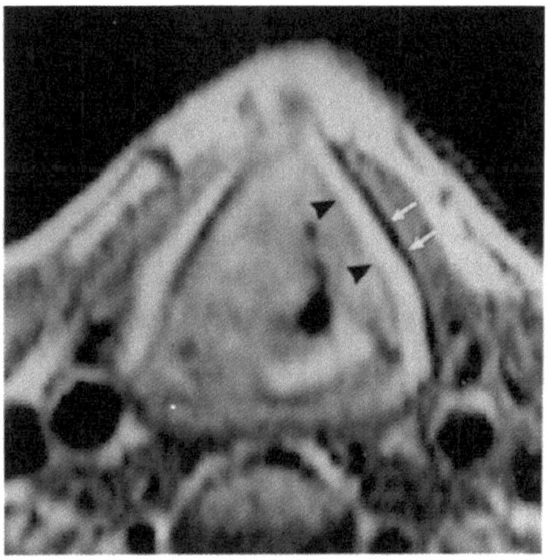

Figure 17. Axial image. Thickening of the outer cortical rim (arrows) and dilution of the inner cortical rim (arrowheads) due to a frequency shift artifact.

frequency exists between hydrogen nuclei bound in water molecules and those bound in lipid molecules. The tissue based frequency shift is misinterpreted upon reconstruction as a difference in spatial location along the frequency-encoded axis. The intrinsic frequency differences appear as spatial shifts in the final image and false edges appear at boundaries where the water-to-fat ratio is significantly different on opposite sides of the boundary. This is particularly notable where fat abuts other tissues. The magnitude of the chemical shift effect depends upon the strength of the main magnetic field and field gradients used, as well as the relative concentration of the two species [5]. Because this effect is proportional to the strength of the main magnetic field, the magnitude of the frequency shift is significantly greater at 1.5 Tesla than at 0.35 Tesla. Fig. 17 shows an example of such a frequency shift artifact. Thickening of the outer cortical rim and dilution of the inner cortical rim may be caused by this kind of artifact.

3.4. *Artifacts due to ferromagnetic implants*

Ferromagnetic implants generate artifacts which depend on the degree of ferromagnetism and the mass of the object. This type of artifact is usually present as a round zone of signal void surrounded by a circumscribed halo of hypersensitivity that fades peripherally. Common sources in the ENT region include stainless steel dental hardware, such as braces, permanent bridges, or root canal pins. Regular tracheal canula does not contain ferromagnetic material. The MR image distortion caused by a magnetic material arises from the disruption of the magnetic field and, therefore, a disruption in the relationship between position and frequency which is necessary for accurate image reconstruction [4]. Consequently, a magnetic object in MRI may cause an artifact, even when it is located outside the slice, since the field lines passing through the region being imaged are distorted [7]. Mostly there is enough distance between the dental prosthesis and the laryngeal area. They never produce artifacts which will interfere with adequate diagnosis of laryngeal cancer.

4. Performance of the laryngeal examination

At my institution, MR imaging is performed with a 0.6 T magnet (Teslacon I; Technicare) and surface coils which surround the neck ventrally and laterally.

The most effective procedure for the reduction of motion artifacts is to educate the patient about the necessity for quiet breathing and limitation of coughing and swallowing. Patients with great difficulty in swallowing, excessive coughing or patients with chronic respiratory disease and/or forced breathing are unsuitable candidates. Objects external to the patient should be removed. The patient is positioned so that the laryngeal airway is as parallel to the tabletop as far as possible.

We begin with a mid- and parasagittal (3 to 5 slices), T1 weighted sequence. This identifies the orientation of the larynx. Axial T1 weighted (SE 310/22 ms), proton density (SE 1500/32 ms) and relatively T2 weighted images (SE 1500/64 ms) are then obtained at corresponding levels. Section thickness is 4 mm, with a 2 mm interslice gap. Four measurements are obtained with T1 weighted and two measurements are obtained with T2 weighted images. Gradient zooming is used to keep the field of view as small as possible. With a 256 × 192 matrix and a field of view of 180 × 180 mm the images have a pixel resolution of 1.4 × 1.0 mm.

References

1. Axel L. Surface coil magnetic resonance imaging. J Comput Assist Tomogr 1984;8:381
2. Hyde JS, Jesmanowicz A, Grist TM, et al. Quadrature detection surface coil. Magn Reson Med 1987;4:179–184.
3. High Resolution Methods Using Local Coils. In: Biomedical Magnetic Resonace Imaging. Principles, Methodology and Application. Wehrli FW, Shaw D. Bruce Kneeland JB,ed. Chapter 5:189–222.
4. Image artifacts and technical limitations. Kelly WM. Chapter 4: 43–82. In: Magnetic resonance imaging of the central nervous system. Brant-Zawadzki M, Norman D. Raven Press, New York, 1986.
5. Artifacts in MR-scanning. In: Elster AD. Magnetic Resonance Imaging. A reference guide and atlas. Lippincott 1986; chapter 5
6. Artifacts. Haacke EM, Bellon EM. Chapter 8:138–159. In: Stark.
7. Kean D. Practical aspects of clinical imaging. In: Kean D, Smith M. Magnetic resonance imaging-principles and applications. William Heineman Medical Books. London. 1986:70–75.

Chapter 6: MR imaging of the normal larynx

by J.A. Castelijns

1. Introduction

The larynx extends from the root of the tongue to the trachea. It projects ventrally between the great vessels of the neck. The skeletal framework of the larynx is formed of cartilages which are connected by ligaments and membranes and moved by a number of muscles. The laryngeal skeleton consist of the hyoid bone, the thyroid, cricoid, the epiglottic and the paired arytenoid cartilages. There are three intralaryngeal compartments: the paired lateral paraglottic spaces and the midline preepiglottic space.

In this chapter MR images of the normal larynx will be demonstrated. In order to gain familiarity with the anatomy of MR images of the larynx it is helpful to use the laryngeal cartilages as landmarks at various axial levels. The cartilages have a unique appearance at each level within the larynx, providing a rapid orientation for any given laryngeal CT or MRI section.

2. MR imaging of laryngeal structures

2.1. *Laryngeal skeleton*

The hyoid bone (Figs. 1, 2b-e, 3a) marks the superior extent of the larynx except for the free-standing epiglottis. This bone is already ossified in infancy and is found on MR images with the typical appearance of bone: a high signal marrow, surrounded by a low signal cortical rim. The hyoid bone has three basic parts: the body and the two greater horns. A zone of low signal intensity, representing a fibrous connection, is present between the body and the two greater horns.

The cricoid cartilage, thyroid cartilage, and the greater part of the arytenoid cartilage consist of hyaline cartilage and are subject to ossification like all hyaline structures. This tends to be an endochondral type of ossification with a true medullary cavity surrounded by a cortical rim. The epiglottic cartilage and the vocal processes of the arytenoids consist of elastic fibrocartilage; this type of cartilage does not generally ossify [1]. On MR SE images non-ossified cartilage (both T1 and T2 weighted images) is seen with intermediate signal intensity. Ossified cartilage is found with a high signal central marrow surrounded by a low signal cortical rim.

The epiglottis (Figs. 1, 3a, b) forms the anterior wall of the laryngeal vestibule. The epiglottis is a thin, multiple perforated elastic cartilage, which

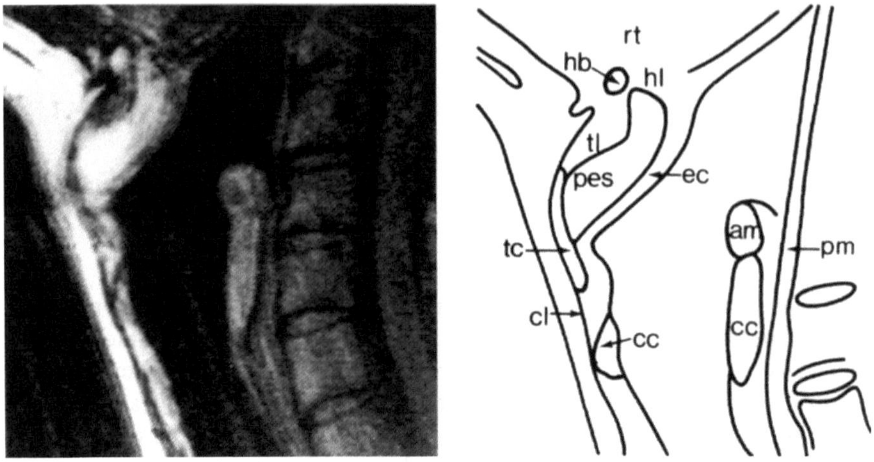

Figure 1. Midsagittal image of a 25–year-old man; field of view: 170 × 170 mm; slice thickness: 5 mm; measurements: 4; SE: 500/50; matrix: 128 × 128. Surface coil. Single slice. For key to abbreviations in scheme see Appendix.

does not generally ossify and is found with intermediate signal intensity on MR images and in high contrast to high signal pre-epiglottic fat. Its inferior extreme, the petiole (Fig. 3c), attaches to the thyroid cartilage via the thyro-epiglottic ligament, at a point just below the thyroid notch. The epiglottis is also attached to the hyoid bone by the hyoepiglottic ligament (Fig. 1). Its free portion projects superiorly just posterior to the valleculae.

The thyroid cartilage is composed of two quadrilateral laminae, 3 cm in height on each side, their anterior borders fuse inferiorly at a median angle, forming the subcutaneous laryngeal prominence ("Adam's apple"). This projection is most distinct at its superior end and is well marked in men but scarcely visible in women. The anterior borders fuse at an angle of about 90 degrees in men and about 120 degrees in women. Immediately above it, the laminae are separated by a V-shaped notch (Fig. 3c), termed the superior thyroid notch. The thyro-epiglottic ligament is attached high in the angle between the laminae; below this, near the midline, the paired vestibular and vocal ligaments and the thyro-arytenoid and vocal muscles are attached in the anterior commissure (Fig. 3d). Posteriorly, the laminae diverge, and the posterior border of each, which is always straight, is elongated as two slender processes: the superior and inferior (Fig. 3e) thyroid cornua. The degree and extent of the ossification of the thyroid cartilage varies. Generally it is

Figure 2. A: Levels at which frontal images were taken. B-F: Frontal images of man; level shown on (A); field of view: 125 × 125 mm; slice thickness: 4 mm; measurements: 2; SE 250/50; matrix 128/128. Surface coil. Single slices. For key to abbreviations in schemes see Appendix.

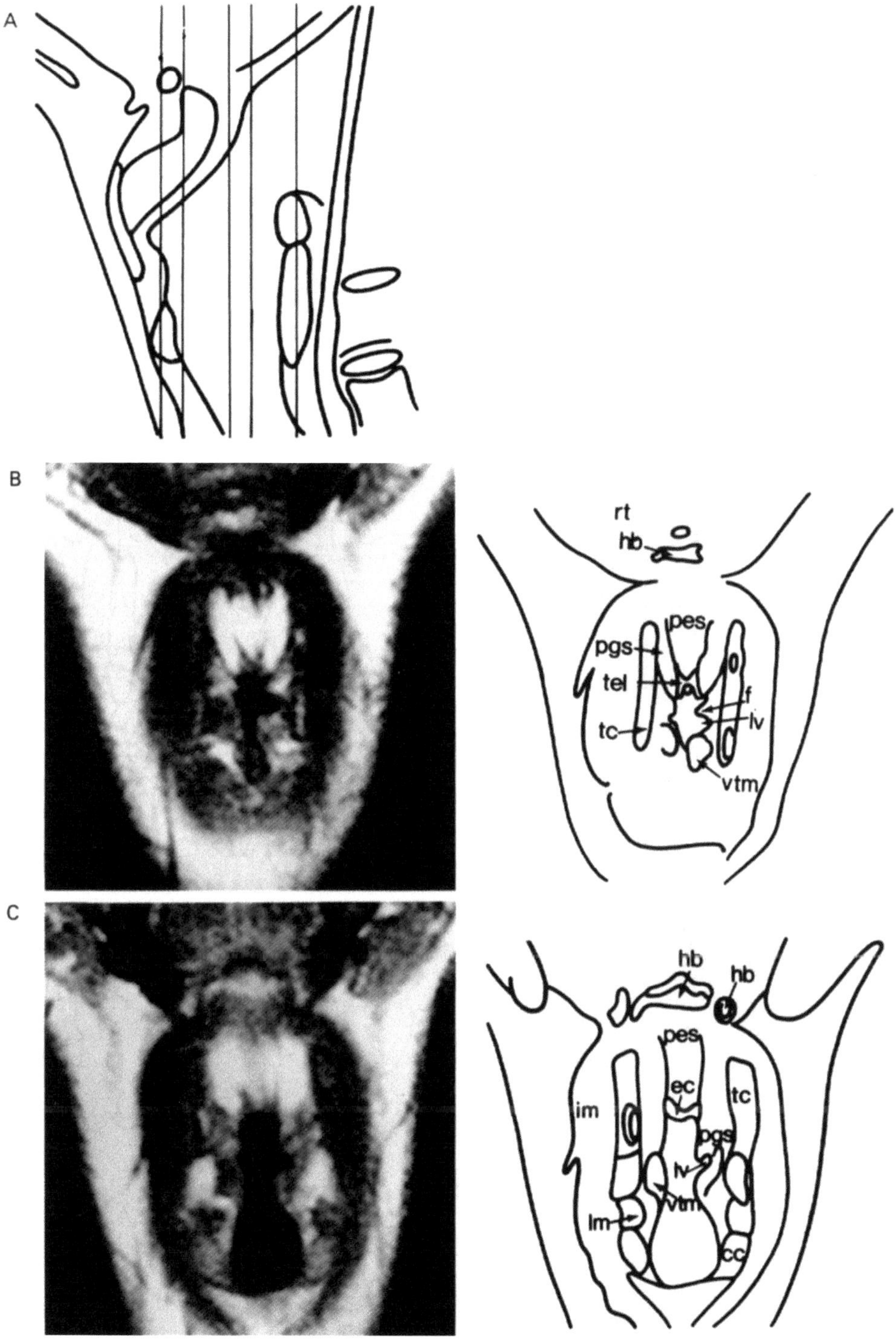
A
B
rt
hb
pes
pgs
tel
tc
f
lv
vtm
C
hb
hb
pes
ec
tc
im
pgs
lv
vtm
lm
cc

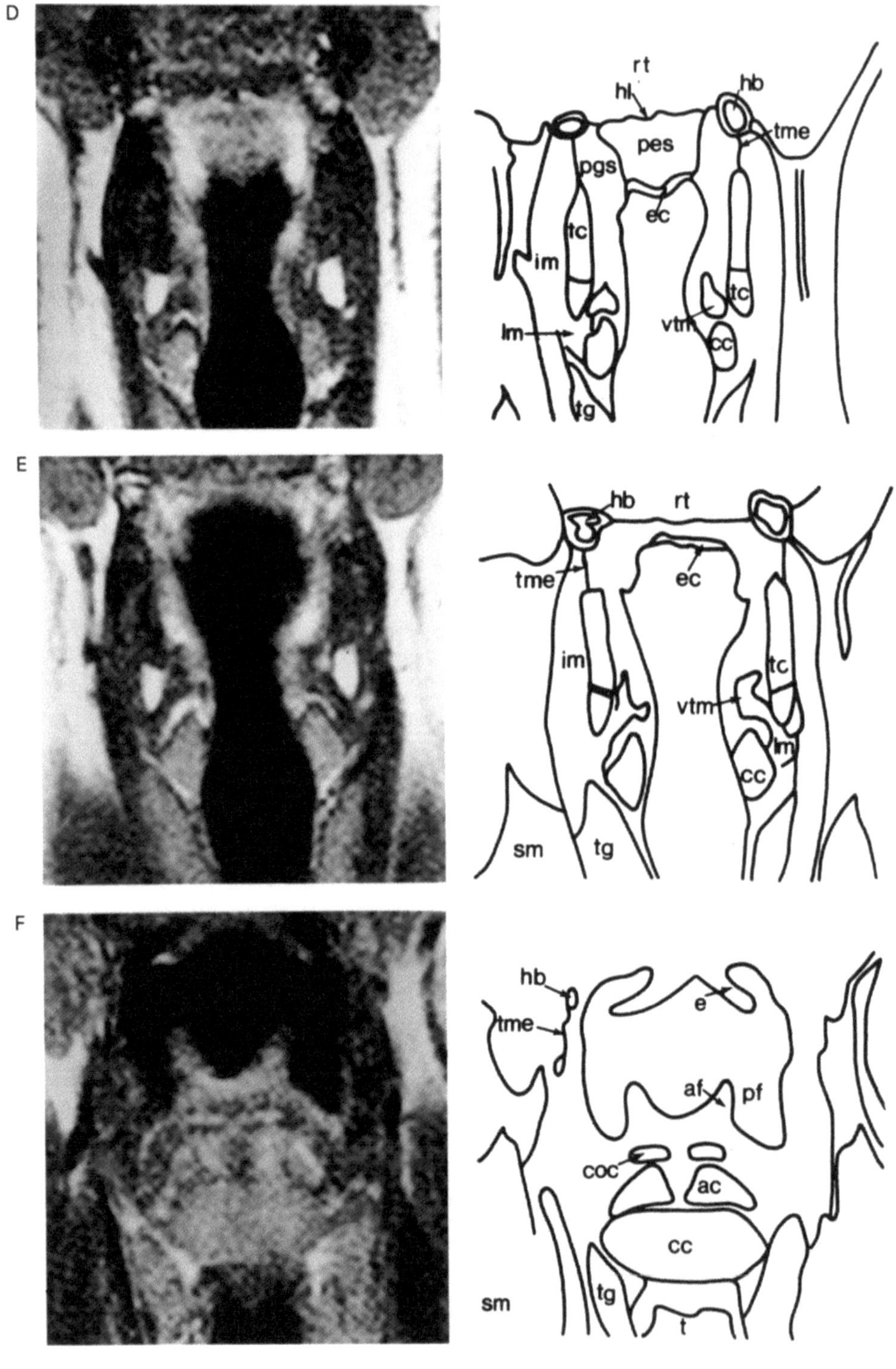
D
rt
hl
hb
tme
pes
pgs
ec
tc
im
tc
vtm
lm
cc
tg
E
hb
rt
tme
ec
im
tc
vtm
lm
cc
sm
tg
F
hb
e
tme
af
pf
coc
ac
cc
sm
tg
t

more ossified in males and moreso with increasing age. Ossification appears to occur mainly in the early twenties and is modified only slightly in the ensuing years. The degree of ossification is greatest in the caudal (Fig. 2d, e) and dorsal portions (Fig. 3c, d) [2]. The inner and outer surfaces do not ossify in a corresponding pattern; the left and right laminae of the thyroid cartilage do not ossify symmetrically (Fig. 2c). Focal areas of ossification are common (Fig. 2c). The MRI signal intensity of the hyaline cartilage is similar to that of the laterally situated infrahyoid muscle (Fig. 2d, e, 3c). Again there is a relative lack of signal from the ossified edges of ossified cartilage and a very high signal from the central fatty marrow.

In quiet respiration the paired arytenoids (Fig. 2f, 3d) are located on the lateral parts of the superior border of the thyroid lamina (Fig. 2f). Each consist of a pyramidal piece with three surfaces, a base, and an apex. The arytenoids consist originally mostly of hyaline cartilage and ossify at an advanced age. The vocal process and the apex consist of elastic cartilage. The signal intensity on MR images varies with the relative degree of ossification.

The cricoid is shaped as a complete signet ring composed of an arch (Fig. 3e) which is narrow in front and measures 5 to 7 mm vertically (Fig. 2c) and a broad lamina posteriorly which is 2 to 3 cm long (Fig. 2f). At the junction of the arch and the lamina, the inferior cornua (Fig. 3e) of the thyroid cartilage articulates with the cricoid at the cricothyroid joints (Fig. 3e). The superior border runs obliquely upward and backward. The facets for the cricoarytenoid joint sit atop the shoulders of the thyroid lamina (Fig. 2f). The cricoid cartilage is frequently well ossified and is then found with the typical MR appearance of bone: a high signal marrow surrounded by a low cortical rim. The signal from non-ossified portions of the cricoid will vary depending on the extent of its ossification.

2.2. *Laryngeal compartments*

Important for the growth and spread of laryngeal cancers are the midline pre-epiglottic space (PES) and the paired lateral paraglottic spaces (PGS) (Fig. 2b, c, d, 3b, c). The PES is seen on MRI with high signal intensity owing to its high fat content. The epiglottic cartilage is seen as an area of relatively low signal intensity just deep to the mucosa (Fig. 1, 2b, c, 3a, b). A zone of decreased signal intensity is mostly visible in the upper part of this space just deep to the epiglottic cartilage (Fig. 1, 2d, 3a). This area of lower signal intensity is produced by the hyoepiglottic ligament. The walls of the PES can be recognized on sagittal images (Fig. 1): the thyrohyoid membrane (and more caudally the thyroid cartilage) as the ventral wall, the epiglottic cartilage as the posterior wall and the hyoepiglottic ligament as the superior wall.

Laterally to the PES, both PGS are situated as shown on the frontal images (Fig. 2b-d). These spaces are bounded laterally by the thyroid and cricoid cartilages with the crico-thyroid ligament and medially by the ventricle, the false vocal cord and the quadrangular membrane [3]. The cricoarytenoid and vocal muscles (Fig. 2d, 3d), lying within the conus elasticus, occupy the inferior portions of the PGS. The two lateral PGSs are filled with loose areolar tissue and the PES is filled with more dense connective tissue, including collagen bundles between mucous glands [3]. The PGS has a high intensity on MR images; the PES has a fairly high intensity. The false cord and the true vocal cord can be identified as two distinct structures, separated by the laryngeal ventricle (Fig. 2c, d). The movable posterior attachments of the true vocal cords are the vocal processes of the arytenoid. The vocal cords meet each other in an immovable anterior commissure, which attaches to the inner perichondrium of the thyroid cartilage (Fig. 2d). On MRI, the vocal cords are normally seen in the abducted position during quiet breathing and are found with intermediate signal intensity. The false vocal cords consist mainly of adipose tissue and therefore show up bright (Fig. 2c) [4].

3. Landmarks

3.1. *Hyoid bone* (*Fig.* 3*a*)

The valleculae may be seen dorsally to the superior part of the hyoid bone.

3.2. *Aryepiglottic fold* (*Fig.* 3*b*)

The laryngeal vestibulum is separated by the aryepiglottic fold from the piriform fossa. Laterally to the piriform fossa and the paraglottic space the upper part of the thyroid lamina may be seen.

3.3. *False vocal cords* (*Fig.* 3*c*)

The thyroid notch is seen 1 cm above the glottic region between the two thyroid laminae. The superior process of the arytenoids may still be visible. The cricoid is not seen at this level. False cords are found with high signal intensity due to fatty tissue. In some patients the sacculus of the laryngeal ventricle may be recognised as an air-filled lucency in the anterior part of the glottic folds.

Figure 3. Axial images of a 32 year old man; field of view: 180 × 180 mm; slice thickness: 5 mm: SE: 250/50; matrix: 128/128. Surface coil. Multiple slice. Levels: A: hyoid bone; B: aryepiglottic fold; C: false vocal cord; D: true vocal cord; E: cricoid cartilage. For key to abbreviations in schemes see Appendix.

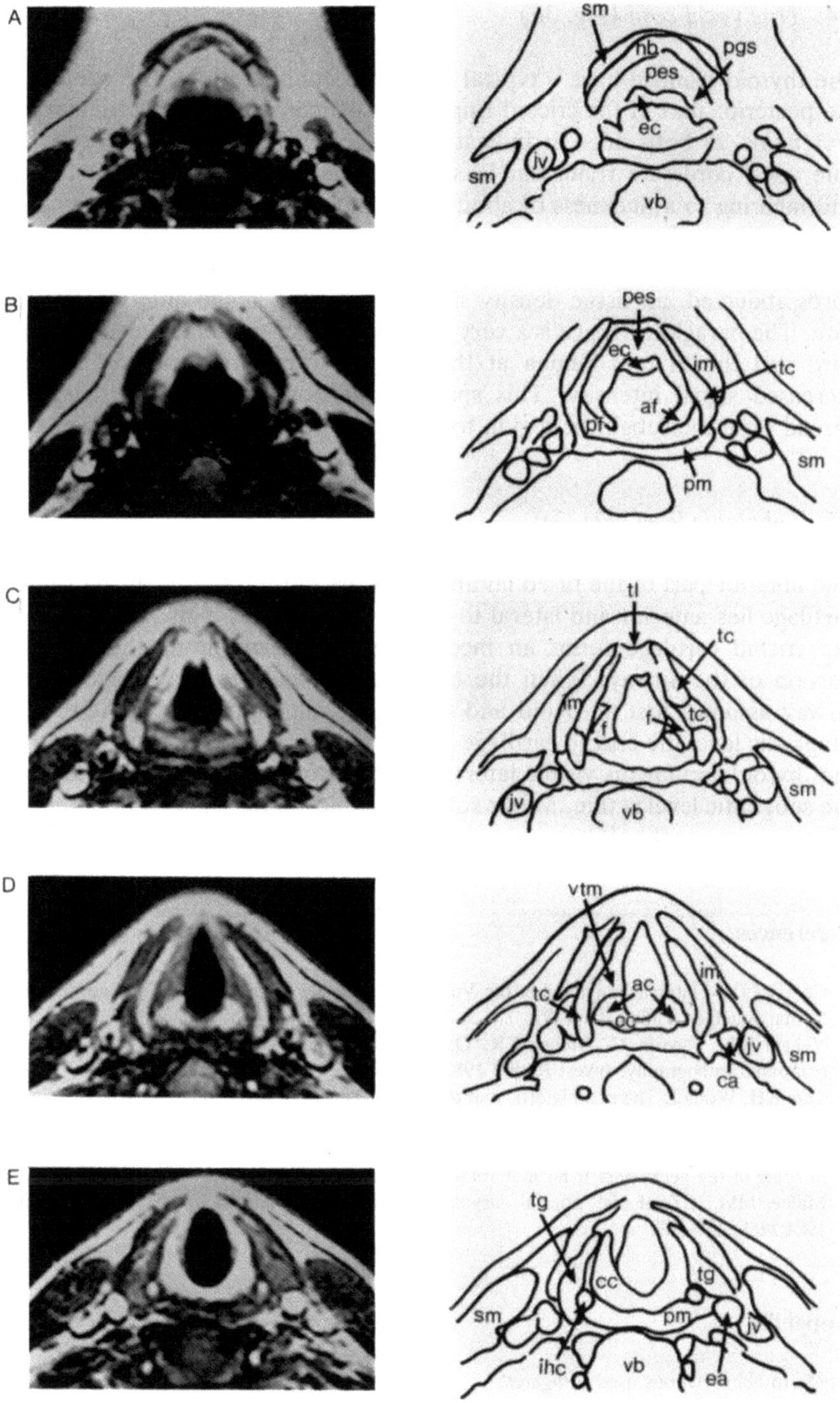
A
sm
hb
pgs
pes
ec
jv
sm
vb
B
pes
ec
im
tc
af
pf
sm
pm
C
tl
tc
im
f
f
tc
sm
jv
vb
D
vtm
im
ac
tc
cc
jv
sm
ca
E
tg
cc
tg
sm
pm
jv
ihc
vb
ea

3.4. *True vocal cord* (*Fig. 3d*)

The thyroid laminae have a typical V-shaped configuration. The contour of the posterior part of the cricoid ring, with two corresponding cartilages, the arytenoids, at both sides, is indicative of the level of the vocal cords. The true vocal cords are triangular in shape, measuring 5 to 6 mm posteriorly and tapering to a thickness of about 1 to 2 mm anteriorly, where they meet the contralateral cord to form the anterior commissure. If the neck is not positioned properly, slight asymmetry will be present. With the true vocal cords abducted, no tissue density should be visible at the anterior commissure. The paraglottic space is a very narrow band of tissue between the vocal cord and the thyroid lamina at this level. It appears as a thin band of increased signal intensity. This space provides a conduit for transglottic spread from the subglottic region to the supraglottic area and vice versa.

3.5. *Subglottic level* (*Fig. 3e*)

The anterior part of the fused laminae appears more rounded as the thyroid cartilage lies anterior and lateral to the cricoid. At this high subglottic level the cricoid cartilage forms an incomplete ring surrounding the posterior portion of the airway. When the transition is made to the subglottis, the airway assumes first an ovoid and then a circular appearance. At the low subglottic level the cricoid cartilage is a complete ring. The cornu inferior of the thyroid cartilage is visible lateral to the cricoid cartilage. The mucosa in the subglottic level is thin. Minor soft tissue thickening suggests the presence of some abnormality [5].

References

1. Chievitz JH. Untersuchungen uber die Verknocherung der menschlichen Kehlknorpel. Arch f Anat Ent Gesch 1882;303–349.
2. Yeager VL, Lawson C, Archer CR. Ossification of laryngeal cartilages as it relates to computed tomography. Invest Radiol 1982;17:11–19.
3. Lam KH, Wong J. The preepiglottic and paraglottic spaces in relation to spread of carcinoma of the larynx. Am J Otolaryngol 1983;4:81–91.
4. Stark DD, Moss AA, Gamsu G, Clark OH, Gooding GA, Webb WR. Magnetic resonance imaging of the neck, part 1: normal anatomy. Radiology 1984;150:447–454.
5. Mafee MM. CT of the normal larynx. In: Radiologic Clinics of Northern America 1984;22(1):251–263.

Appendix

Guide to abbreviations used in figures:
ac, arytenoid cartilage; af, aryepiglottic fold; am, arytenoid muscles: ca, common carotid artery;

cc, cricoid cartilage: cl, cricothyroid ligament; coc, corniculate cartilage; e, epiglottis, ec, epiglottic cartilage; f, false vocal cord; hb, hyoid bone; hl, hyoepiglottic ligament; shc, superior horn of cartilage; ihc, inferior horn of cartilage; im, infrahyoid muscles; jv, internal jugular vein; lm, lateral cricoarytenoid muscle; lv, laryngeal ventricle; pcm, posterior cricoarytenoid muscle; pes, preepiglottic space; pf, piriform fossa; pgs, paraglottic space; pm, constrictor pharyngis muscle: rt, root of the tongue; sm, sternocleidomastoid muscle; sv, superior laryngeal vein; tc, thyroid cartilage; tel, thyroepiglottic ligament; tg, thyroid gland; tl, thyrohyoid ligament; tme, thyrohyoid membrane; vb, vertebral body; vn, vagus nerve; vtm, vocalis/thyroarytenoid muscle.

Chapter 7: MR imaging of laryngeal cancer

Authors: J.A. Castelijns (M.D.) (1)
M.C. Kaiser (M.D.) (1)
J. Valk (M.D.) (1)
G.J. Gerritsen (M.D.) (2)
A.H. van Hattum (M.D.) (3)
G.B. Snow (M.D.) (2)

(1) Department of Radiology
(2) Department of Otolaryngology/
Head and Neck Surgery
(3) Pathology

Institution: Free University Hospital
Amsterdam
The Netherlands

Abstract

Forty-four consecutive patients with laryngeal carcinomas presenting at different stages of the disease were investigated by magnetic resonance (MR) imaging. Twelve patients (six with primary lesions and six with recurrent tumors) underwent laryngectomy, and the macro- and microscopic appearance of the sliced specimens were correlated with MR imaging. In the remaining patients surgery was not performed, and MR results were compared with the laryngoscopic findings. Cancerous tissue was seen on T1 weighted images as a homogeneous mass of intermediate signal intensity, slightly higher than infrahyoid muscles. The MR examinations failed mainly in patients with tumor recurrence who had undergone previous radiation treatment.

1. Introduction

In the past, clinical examination and conventional radiological techniques (tomography and laryngography) were the diagnostic tools available for preoperative evaluation of the location and extent of carcinomas of the larynx and hypopharynx. Computed tomography added the ability to demonstrate intralaryngeal pathways of tumor spread, such as submucosal tumor growth and gross cartilage destruction. This information is very useful for staging advanced carcinomas of the larynx and hypopharynx and for deciding whether radiation therapy or surgery is indicated [1].

Nevertheless, CT of the larynx has its limitations, especially in determining early cartilage invasion and in trying to provide a three-dimensional representation of pathology. Magnetic resonance (MR) imaging displays greater soft tissue detail in axial, frontal and sagittal planes [2]. From previously reported studies [3–7] it appears that MR shows the anatomy of the larynx, in particular the intrinsic laryngeal musculature and the intralaryngeal compartments, with excellent detail and soft tissue definition.

To evaluate how well MR can display the larynx and its surrounding structures, we compared the results of MR imaging with pathological specimens following laryngectomy or with laryngoscopic findings when radiation treatment had to be carried out. Seven representative cases out of a series of 44 consecutive MR investigations of the larynx have been selected in which correlation with pathological specimens and laryngoscopic findings has been emphasized.

2. Materials and methods

Forty-four consecutive patients presenting with laryngeal carcinomas at different TNM stages have been investigated by MR imaging. Thirty patients had primary and 14 had recurrent disease after irradiation treatment. Primary carcinomas included six supraglottic, 19 glottic, one subglottic and four piriform sinus tumors. We selected the most appropriate pulse sequences and the most adequate patient and coil positioning on the basis of earlier experience with MRI in 16 patients who were not included in this study. Images were acquired with a 0.6 T superconductive system (Technicare) using a half saddle-shaped surface coil placed around the anterior aspect of the neck as a receiver antenna. Routinely, a three slice technique in a sagittal plane spin echo (SE) 200/38 was obtained. The T1 weighted images in the frontal (SE 300/38) and axial planes (SE 400/38) were centered on the lesion as seen on the midline sagittal ("Scout") image. The T2 weighted images (SE 1500/38, SE 1500/76) were obtained in the axial plane. The slice thickness used was 4 mm with 3 mm gaps. Four measurements were obtained with T1 weighted and two measurements with T2 weighted images. Gradient zooming was used to keep the field of view as small as possible (20 × 20 cm). With a 256 × 192 matrix the images had a pixel resolution of 0.8 × 1.0 mm.

Twelve patients (six with primary lesions and six with recurrent tumors) underwent laryngectomy and the specimens were obtained for sectioning. The specimens were fixed in 4% formaldehyde, then decalcified by submersion in Kristensen's solution for 2 weeks. According to the recommendations of Michaels and Gregor [8], axial slices with a 4 mm thickness were cut parallel to the plane of the axial MR slices. All slices were photographed and parts of the slices were processed for microscopic examination. A comparison was performed between axial MR images, macroscopic sections, and microscopic findings in order to identify tumor tissue and to evaluate whether infiltration of cartilage existed.

3. Case reports

Case 1

A 59–year old man complained of hoarseness, swallowing difficulties, and bilateral otalgia of a few months' duration. Laryngoscopy showed an ulcerating mass on the laryngeal aspect of the epiglottis. This mass was mainly left-sided but extended to the right. The left aryepiglottic fold was involved, but the arytenoid seemed to be intact. The tumor was staged as a T1N0 supraglottic lesion. An axial T1 weighted image of the larynx at the level of the aryepiglottic fold (Fig. 1a) clearly demonstrated thickening of the left aryepiglottic fold with compression of the piriform sinus. The pre-epiglottic space (PES) was infiltrated and enlarged by a mass with abnormal signal

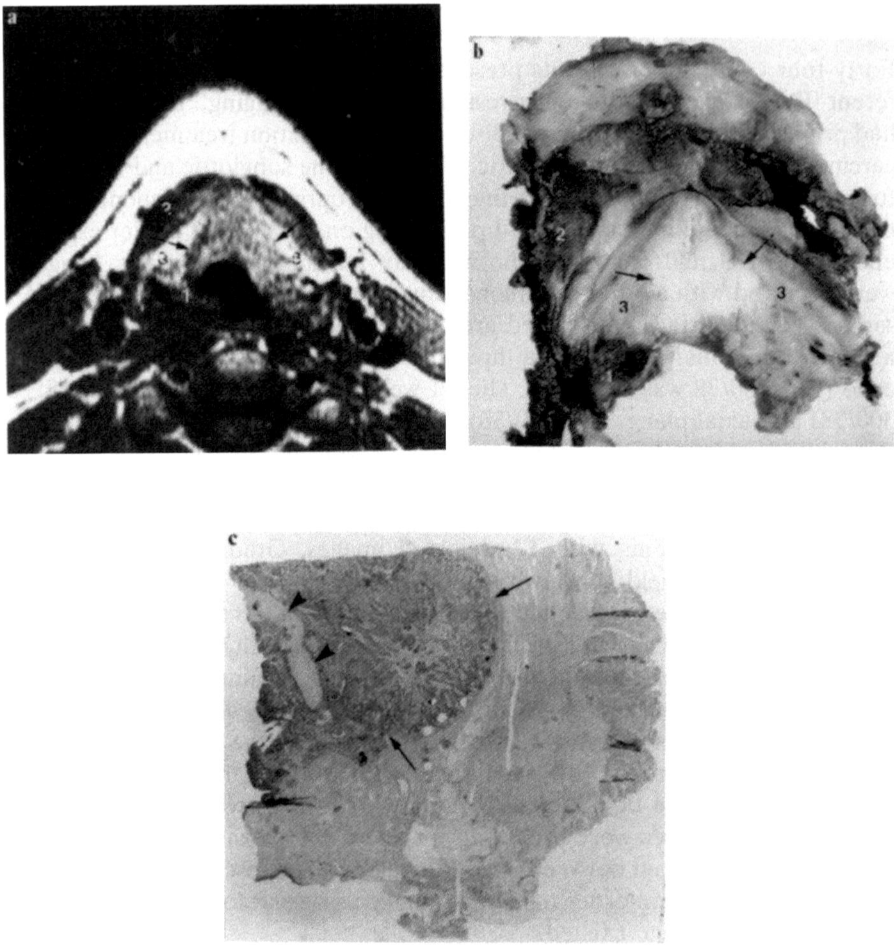

Figure 1. Case 1. Patient with T1N0 supraglottic tumor. A: Axial image (SE 400/38) at level of aryepiglottic fold (1) demonstrates tumor (arrows) in preepiglottic space with a slightly higher signal intensity than the infrahyoid muscles (2) but definitely lower signal intensity than fatty tissue within paraglottic space (3). B: Axial macroscopic section corresponding to (A). Tumor is recognized as a white structure (arrows) with similar contours and a topographic relation to neighboring structures as shown by MR. The numbers are identical in (A and B). C: Microscopic section corresponding to left posterior quadrant of (B) outlines nonossified epiglottic cartilage with obvious tumor invasion (arrowheads) locates within tumor tissue (arrows).

intensity, higher than the signal intensity of muscular tissue. The nonossified epiglottic cartilage could not be identified within the surrounding tumor.

A section of the postoperative specimen at the corresponding level showed that the contour of the tumor corresponded to the lesion as outlined by MR. This section also confirmed the MRI finding of a compressed paraglottic space (PGS), normally filled by fatty tissues (Fig. 1b). On histopathological examination the nonossified cartilage within the tumor tissue showed tumor invasion (Fig. 1c).

Case 2

A 62-year-old man complained of long-standing hoarseness. Laryngoscopy showed an ulcerating tumor, originating from the posterior aspect of the right laryngeal ventricle. This mass extended superiorly into the posterior part of the false cord, which was displaced cranially. The mass also extended

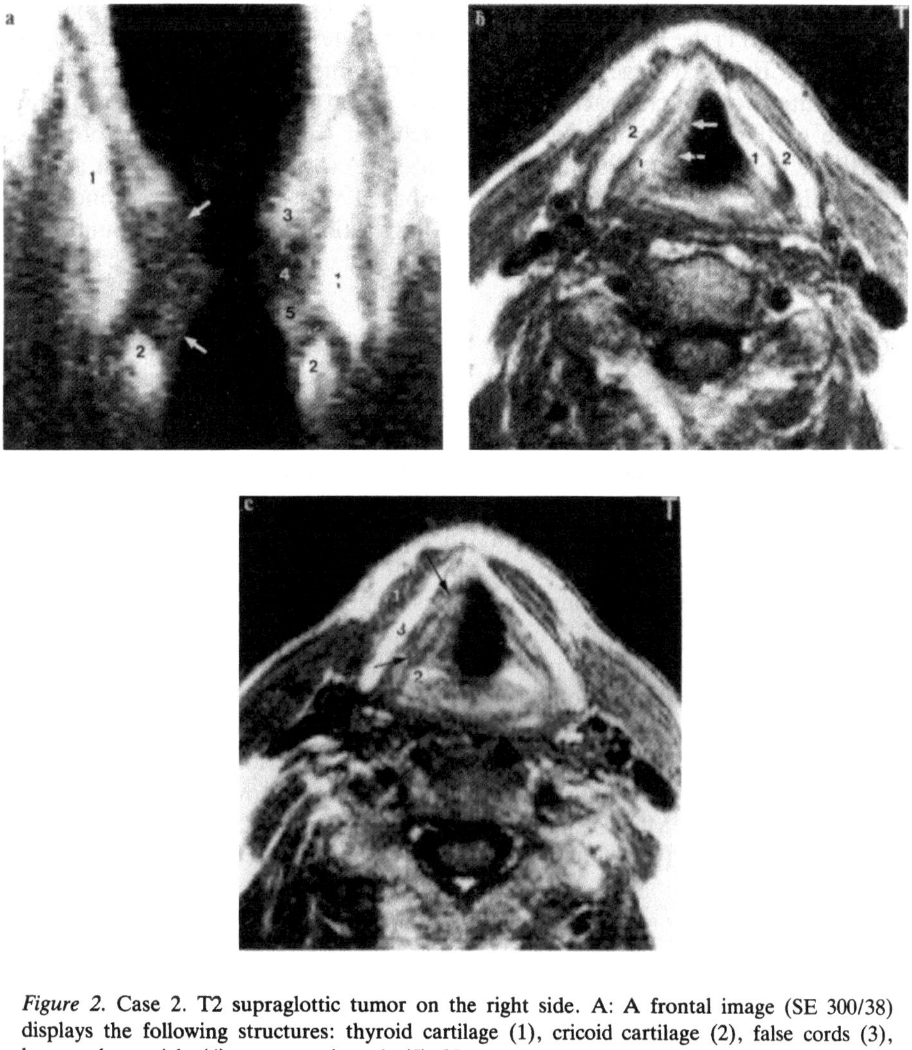

Figure 2. Case 2. T2 supraglottic tumor on the right side. A: A frontal image (SE 300/38) displays the following structures: thyroid cartilage (1), cricoid cartilage (2), false cords (3), laryngeal ventricle (4), true vocal cords (5). Note area of intermediate signal intensity on the right side due to tumor tissue (arrows). B: Axial slice (SE 400/38) shows false cord (1), and ossified thyroid cartilage (2). Tumor compresses right vocal cord laterally (arrows). C: Axial image (SE 400/38) at level of true vocal cords. The tumor is shown as a sharply defined mass (arrows) having a slightly higher signal intensity than the infrahyoid muscles (1). It is contiguous to arytenoid cartilage (2) and the thyroid cartilage (3).

caudally into the true vocal cord. The tumor was clinically staged as a T2 supraglottic lesion. The T1 weighted images in the frontal plane showed an intermediate intensity mass on the right side. The region of the true and false vocal cords was invaded by the process, while fat tissue of the right vocal cord was displaced upward (Fig. 2a). Axial MR slices showed the false vocal cords as structures of high signal intensity. A mass of intermediate intensity was demonstrated at the posterior edge of the right false cord (Fig. 2b). At the level of the true vocal cord, this intermediate signal intensity mass, located in the PGS, was adjacent to the arytenoid and thyroid cartilages (Fig. 2c). Both cartilages were ossified; bone marrow was seen with high signal intensity and compact bone with low signal intensity. The cortical rim of the cartilage was intact, and we concluded that there was no obvious cartilage invasion. As T2 tumors are treated by irradiation treatment at our hospital, MR images could only be compared with laryngoscopic findings; correlation between the results of both diagnostic modalities was found.

Case 3

A 58–year-old man presented with hoarseness and soreness of the throat. Laryngoscopy showed a tumor invading the medial, lateral and anterior walls of the right piriform sinus, but the floor of the piriform sinus appeared to be uninvolved. Axial T1 weighted MR scans at the level of the thyroid notch showed a swelling of the anterior, medial and lateral walls of the right piriform sinus. This lesion had intermediate signal intensity and could not be differentiated from surrounding tissues (Fig. 3a). Extension of the lesion in the direction of the infrahyoid muscles was shown. Although this tumor also extended dorsolaterally, invasion of the carotid artery could be excluded by MRI. Macroscopic section at the level of the thyroid notch showed the tumor corresponding to the region of intermediate signal intensity on MRI. The mass extended along the ventral side of the superior horn, passed over the superior edge of the thyroid cartilage, and spread toward the infrahyoid muscles (Fig. 3b). Microscopic sections showed tumor involvement of the infrahyoid muscles (Fig. 3c).

Case 4

A 72–year-old man complained of progressively increasing hoarseness over a period of one year. Dyspnea with inspiratory stridor and pain during swallowing developed within the preceding few weeks. Laryngoscopy showed a transglottic tumor on the left extending into the anterior commissure. Fixation of the vocal cords was found and the tumor was staged as T3NO. Axial MR slices at the level of the true vocal cord showed a large homogene-

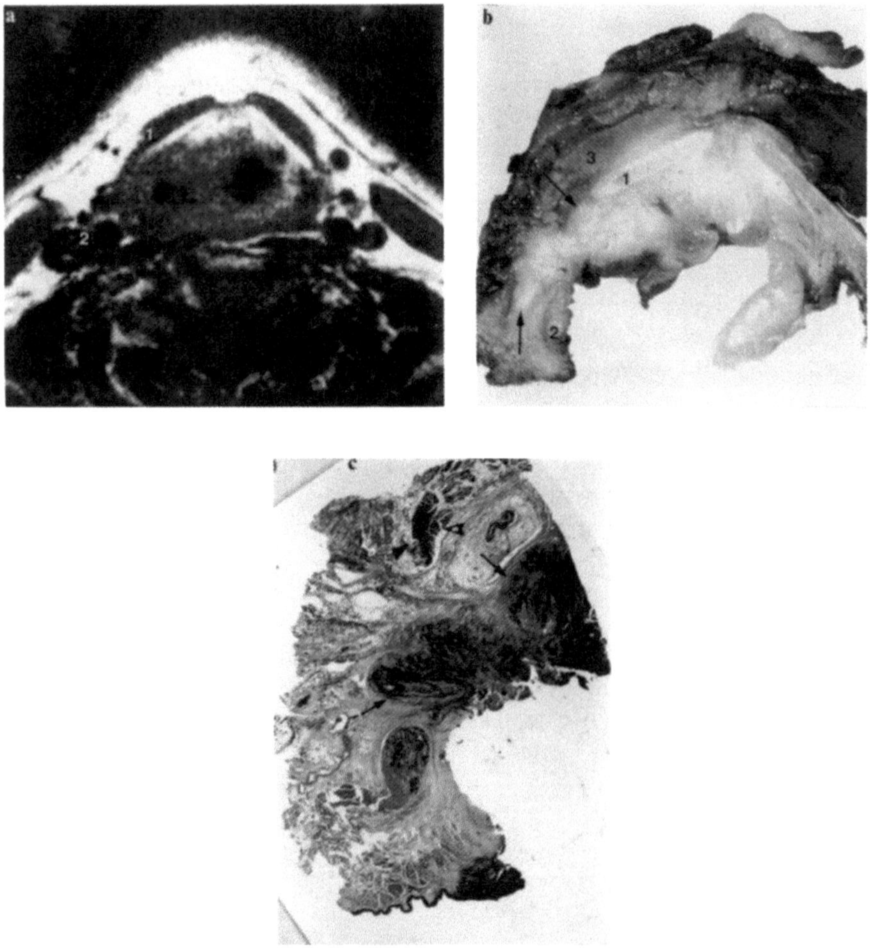

Figure 3. Case 3. Patient with tumor of piriform sinus. A: Axial scan (SE 400/38) at level of thyroid notch displays large area with intermediate signal intensity extending toward the right infrahyoid muscles (1) and the carotid sheath (2). B: Macroscopic section at corresponding level shows the tumor (arrows), the lamina of the thyroid cartilage (1), and its superior horn (2), and the infrahyoid muscles (3). C: Microscopic study of the right posterior quadrant of (B). Tumor (arrows) approaches the infrahyoid muscles (arrowheads).

ous area of intermediate signal intensity located within the left PGS and the anterior commissure region. This area had higher signal intensity than the neighboring infrahyoid muscles (Fig. 4a). Anteriorly, the tumor invaded the thyroid cartilage and extended into the prelaryngeal infrahyoid muscles (Fig. 4a and b). Posteriorly, the intermediate intensity area extended into the right arytenoid and the cricoid lamina (Fig. 4a). A midsagittal scan outlined the

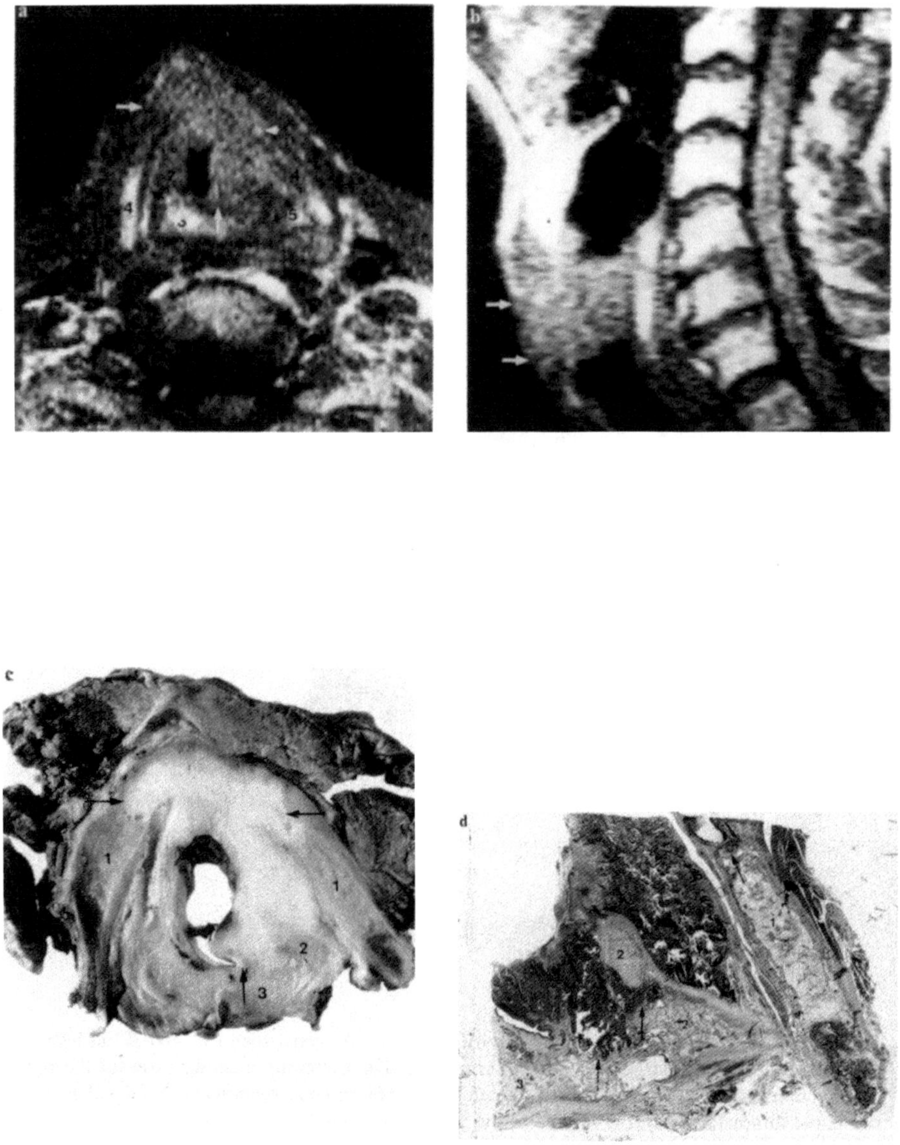

Figure 4. Case 4. T3N0 transglottic tumor. A: Axial image (SE 400/38) at the glottic level shows tumor (arrows) with a slightly higher signal intensity than infrahyoid (1), vocal, and thyroarytenoid muscles (2). Gross destruction of the cricoid (3), the thyroid cartilage (4), and left arytenoid cartilage (5) is present. B: Sagittal section (SE 200/38) shows prelaryngeal (arrows) and craniocaudal extension of tumor extending from the glottic to the low subglottic level. C: Macroscopic section corresponds to (A). Neoplastic invasion of cartilage (arrows) was confirmed: the thyroid (1), the left arytenoid (2), and the cricoid (3) showed obvious tumor invasion. D: Microscopic examination of the left posterior quadrant of specimen (C) confirmed tumor invasion (arrows) of the thyroid (1), left arytenoid (2), and the cricoid (3) cartilages.

large homogeneous mass extending from the glottic level to the low subglottic area. Macroscopic sections at the corresponding levels confirmed MR findings (Fig. 4c).

Microscopic examination demonstrated invasion of the three cartilages on the left (Fig. 4d) and prelaryngeal extension with invasion of the infrahyoid muscles (not illustrated).

Case 5

A 75–year-old man complained of hoarseness, dyspnea, and coughing over a period of 8 months. Laryngoscopy revealed a solid glottic process on the right with submucosal extension to the supraglottic level. The false cord, the laryngeal ventricle, and the aryepiglottic fold were affected. A small ulceration was seen within the anterior commissure. Clinically, the tumor was staged as T3NO. Figure 5a is an axial MR slice, displaying enlargement of the right PGS just above the glottic level. The entire PGS contained intermediate signal tumor extending toward the anterior commissure. The thyroid cartilage and the right arytenoid were still intact. The corresponding macroscopic section revealed that right PGS was invade by tumor (Fig. 5b). Histopathological study confirmed that cartilage invasion was not present (not illustrated).

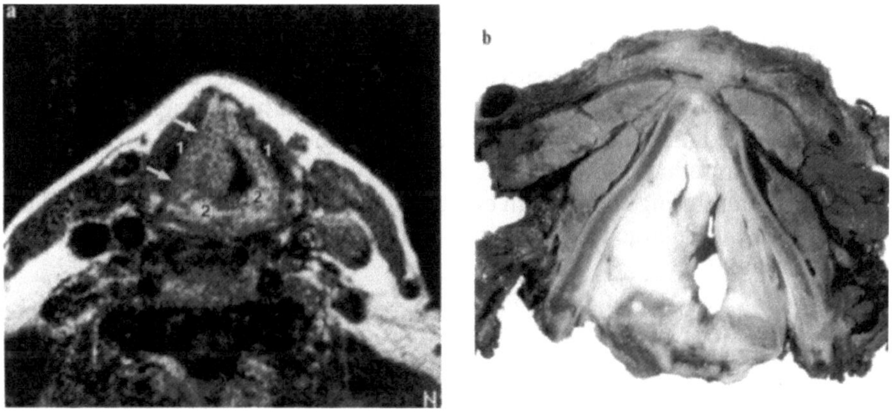

Figure 5. Case 5. T3N0 transglottic larynx carcinoma. A: An axial MR image (SE 400/38) at level of thyroid notch shows the thyroid cartilage with intermediate signal intensity since most of it is not yet ossified (1). The ossified arytenoids (2) have high signal intensity. Tumor (arrows) fills the right paraglottic space (PGS) and approaches the thyroid and arytenoid cartilages but no cartilage invasion was apparent. B: Macroscopic section at same level as (A). Tumor is seen as a white tissue mass in the right PGS. Cartilage invasion was excluded.

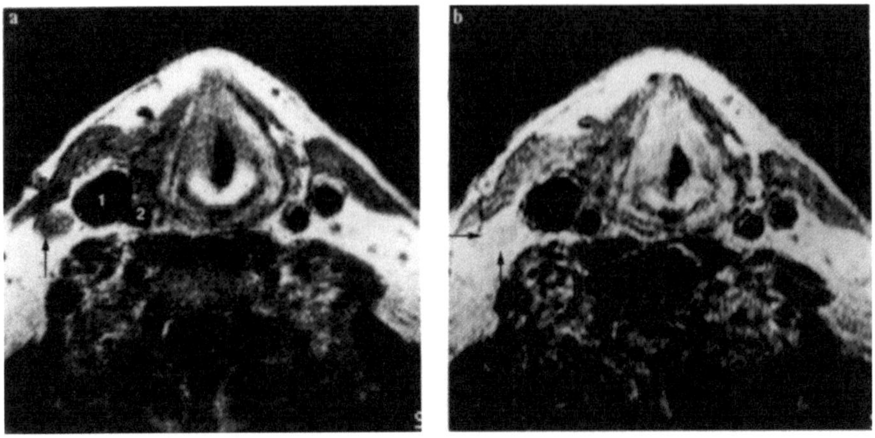

Figure 6. Case 6. T4 piriform sinus tumor with intracapsular lymph node spread. A: T1–weighted image (SE 400/38) demonstrates enlarged lymph node with an intermediate signal intensity (arrow) on the right, easily differentiated from the jugular vein (1), carotid artery (2), and the fatty tissues within the carotid sheath. B: T2–weighted slice (SE 1500/76) visualizes the malignant node (arrows) with high signal intensity optimizing its differentiation from vascular structures.

Case 6

A 65–year-old man complained about soreness of the throat and dyspnea over 6 months. A progressive swelling of the right neck over 3 months was noted, due to a pathological lymph node. Laryngoscopy revealed a T4 piriform sinus tumor. A T1 weighted image (Fig. 6a) showed the lymph node with an intermediate signal intensity. This node had a smooth contour and was easily distinguished from surrounding fatty tissue. A T2 weighted axial scan at the corresponding level showed the node with higher signal intensity. Although the contrast definition between the enlarged node and surrounding fatty tissue was reduced, delineation from vascular structures became optimal (Fig. 6b). Total laryngectomy with en bloc neck dissection revealed malignant spread into the enlarged node, but extranodular extension was not shown (not illustrated).

Case 7

A 66–year-old man complained of swallowing difficulties, hoarseness and left-sided otalgia. A supraglottic carcinoma, staged as T4N3, was found by laryngoscopy. A 2.5 cm lymph node was palpated in the left subdigastric region. Axial MR scans at the supraglottic level confirmed the presence of a primary carcinoma in the left aryepiglottic fold. The T1 weighted images demonstrated the pathological lymph node as an irregularly shaped soft tissue mass of intermediate signal intensity, easily differentiated from surrounding

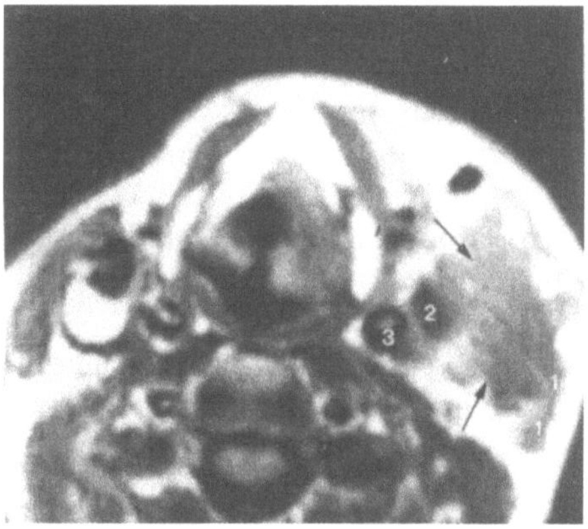

Figure 7. Case 7. Patient with supraglottic tumor and extracapsular lymph node spread. Axial MR delineates lymphatic invasion (arrows) with intermediate signal intensity in comparison to sternocleidomastoid muscle (1), which has a relatively lower signal intensity. Metastatic spread into surrounding fat and muscle is obvious on the left. Internal jugular vein (2) and carotid artery (3) are well displayed.

fat. Infiltration of the sternocleidomastoid muscle was present, muscular tissue having a slightly lower signal intensity than metastatic lymph node spread (Fig. 7). Total laryngectomy with en bloc neck dissection demonstrated lymph node metastasis with extranodular spread into surrounding fat and muscular tissue, confirming our preoperative MR findings (not illustrated).

4. Discussion

MR imaging of laryngeal carcinomas is difficult due to these patients' dyspnea, coughing and mucous secretion. Our study has nevertheless shown that, by using shorter scanning times, MR was capable of providing good diagnostic results in almost all the cases. Further improvement of MR results may be achieved by administering drugs to inhibit coughing and mucous secretion or by sedating the patient. In our experience MR examinations failed mainly in patients with recurrent tumors after radiation treatment, partially due to their poor clinical condition and motion artifacts (14 cases). Even when the MR images in those cases were of technically good quality, distinction between residual of recurrent tumor, radiation fibrosis, and edema was not possible. On T1 weighted images the intralaryngeal soft tissue structures could be demonstrated with intermediate signal intensity, whereas on T2 weighted images they were seen with high signal intensity. The lack of tissue differentiation by MR in cases of tumor recurrences is in agreement with the experience of Worthman et al. [7] but is contradictory to statements made by Glazer et al. [9], who claimed that, in the mediastinum, T2 weighted images (SE 1500/90) were helpful in distinguishing recurrent tumor from radiation fibrosis. Since T1 weighted images accurately assess the extension of primary laryngeal cancer, we stress their importance in demonstrating tumor invasion into different areas: (a) intralaryngeal region (PES, PGS, subglottic region, anterior commisure); (b) laryngeal cartilages; (c) extralaryngeal structures (piriform sinus, infrahyoid muscles, carotid sheath, lymph nodes).

The T1 weighted images in the three planes displayed the three intralaryngeal compartments (both PGS and PES) with high contrast and all bordering structures were clearly shown [5, 6]. In the three illustrated specimens of primary laryngeal carcinomas the topographic relation between tumor and surrounding structures corresponded well with MR findings. Site, extension and contour of the tumor mass as shown by axial MR corresponded to the actual configuration of the lesions seen on specimens (Figs. 1, 4 and 5). Extension of submucosal tumor in the intralaryngeal compartments was well defined by axial MR. At the supraglottic level tumor tissue was seen as a homogeneous mass of intermediate signal intensity, lower than the signal intensity of fat. By contrast, on the level of the true vocal cords, tumor has a relatively higher signal intensity than fat and a slightly higher signal intensity than the vocal and thyroarytenoid muscles. Subglottic and craniocaudal extension is well displayed in the frontal plane (Fig. 2a). To perform a supraglottic laryngectomy a 3 to 5 mm tumor-free margin above the level of the anterior commissure should exist and the cartilages should not be invaded [1, 10]. Sagittal MR images are most appropriate for the assessment of this tumor-free margin. In agreement with the literature we also found that this scanning plane is helpful in demonstrating or excluding infiltration of the tongue base, hyoid bone, and prelaryngeal region (Fig. 4b) [6].

Diagnosis of cartilage invasion has a major therapeutic impact. If present, perichondritis and necrosis with subsequent severe edema are likely to occur as complications following radiation therapy, and the incidence of tumor recurrence is also significantly higher [1]. The cricoid, thyroid, and greater part of the arytenoid cartilages are composed of hyaline cartilage, which is subject to ossification. The epiglottic cartilage and both vocal processes are composed of yellow fibrocartilage, which does not ossify [11]. If malignant invasion of hyaline cartilage occurs, it remains confined to its ossified components in most cases [12, 13]. Ossified cartilage, composed of compact bone surrounding marrow, has a typical three-layer appearance (Fig. 2, 3a, and 4a). Invasion into this cartilage can be recognized as an area of intermediate signal intensity interrupting the typical three-layer appearance (Fig. 4a). Gross cartilage invasion is routinely shown by axial MR. Nonossified epiglottic cartilage is normally shown with high contrast compared with neighbouring fat [5]. When cancer invades this area, the cartilage cannot be identified within tumor tissue by MRI (Fig. 1a).

In the two cases of the piriform sinus tumors, correlation between MRI and specimens was less evident. Demonstration of infiltration into extralaryngeal soft tissue structures (i.e. infrahyoid muscles, carotid sheath, and lymph nodes) is important in determining margins of surgical resection. Axial images may provide evidence of malignant invasion of the infrahyoid muscles (Figs. 3a and 4a); extension into the carotid sheath can be demonstrated or excluded because contrast between fat within the carotid sheath and tumor is increased (Fig. 3a). The contour of pathological lymph nodes is also well defined and contrast medium administration is not needed (Figs. 6 and 7). If lymph nodes are irregularly outlined, extranodal spread should be suspected (Fig. 7). If nodes are smoothly bordered on axial MR images (Fig. 6), the probability of extranodal spread decreases. Three-dimensional T1 weighted MR imaging permits calculation of the volume of the tumor mass, which is one of the most important criteria in establishing a prognosis concerning the efficiency of irradiation treatment. The T2 weighted images appear to be inappropriate for the display of primary tumors, since tumor tissue is visualized less homogeneously and the signal-to-noise ratio of the image is decreased [6]. Tumor and reactive edema both have high signal intensity and cannot be separated by MRI. The T2 weighted images are useful in detecting pathological lymph nodes, which have higher signal intensity and are more easily differentiated from vascular structures (Fig. 6) [14].

5. Conclusions

In the analysis of our series of 30 patients with primary laryngeal tumors we came to the following conclusions:

1. In seven cases with tumors clinically staged as T1aNO glottic, MRI showed either no abnormalities or no obvious pathological findings. For this reason we think that MRI is not indicated in those cases.
2. In glottic tumors clinically staged as T1bNO glottic (three cases) and T2NO glottic (five cases) lesions, axial T1 weighted MR images showed at one level an abnormal area of homogeneous intermediate signal intensity. Important information concerning tumor extension toward the arytenoid and thyroid cartilages was obtained. Cartilage invasion could not be excluded or confirmed by MRI in these relatively small lesions. Further studies including histopathological correlation will be needed for this purpose.
3. Axial MRI slices of more advanced glottic tumors (three T3NO and one T4NO) routinely demonstrated a well defined homogeneous region of intermediate signal intensity. Moreover, it was possible to show cartilage invasion and infiltration of infrahyoid muscles. In these cases frontal MR

images showed obvious asymmetry between the right and left PGS so that the cranial and caudal extensions of the lesions were more precisely outlined.
4. In our experience with six cases of supraglottic tumors, sagittal MR images helped to define the distance of the abnormal signal intensity area to the root of the tongue, to the anterior commissure and to the hyoid bone.
5. In four cases of piriform sinus tumors there was an obvious difference of signal intensity between the pathological area and the fat within the carotid sheath. Information about the relationship of the lesion to the infrahyoid and sternocleidomastoid muscles as well as about possible extension into the posterior hypopharyngeal wall could be obtained.
6. On T1 weighted images pathological lymph nodes were seen with intermediate intensity, whereas T2 weighted images showed an increased intensity.

Magnetic resonance imaging may play a major role in the diagnostic workup of primary laryngeal tumors. Although scanning times had to be shortened due to the rather poor clinical condition of the patients, we obtained mostly high quality T1 weighted images in patients with primary disease. It is possible to demonstrate submucosal tumor extension in the PES and PGS, cartilage invasion, and enlarged pathological lymph nodes. In our experience MRI failed in patients with recurrent tumor following radiation treatment.

References

1. Gerritsen GJ. Computed tomography and laryngeal cancer Academic thesis. Amsterdam: Free University of Amsterdam, 1984.
2. Valk J, MacLean C, Algra PR. The clinical application of NMR tomography. In: Valk J, ed. Basic principles of nuclear magnetic resonance imaging. Amsterdam: Elsevier, 1985:115–140.
3. Lufkin RB, Larsson SG, Hanafee WN. Work in progress: NMR anatomy of the larynx and the tongue base. Radiology 1983;148:173–175.
4. Stark DD, Moss AA, Gamsu G, Clark OH, Gooding GA, Webb WR. Magnetic resonance imaging of the neck. Part 1: normal anatomy. Radiology 1984;150:447–452.
5. Castelijns JA, Doornbos J, Verbeeten B Jr., Vielvoye GJ, Bloem JL. MR imaging of the normal larynx. J Comput Assist Tomogr 1985;9:919–925.
6. Lufkin RB, Hanafee WN, Wortham D, Hoover L. Larynx and hypopharynx: MR imaging with surface coils. Radiology 1986;158:747–754.
7. Wortham DG, Hoover LA, Lufkin RB, Fu YS. Magnetic resonance imaging of the larynx: a correlation with histologic sections. Otolaryngol Head Neck 1986;94:123–133.
8. Michaels L, Gregor RT. Examination of the larynx in the histopathology laboratory. J Clin Pathol 1980;33:705–710.
9. Glazer HS, Lee JK, Levitt RG, et al. Radiation fibrosis: differentiation from recurrent tumor by MR imaging. Radiology 1985;156:721–726.
10. Mancuso AA, Hanafee WN. Larynx and hypopharynx. In: Stamathis G, ed. Computed tomography and magnetic resonance of the head and neck. Baltimore: Williams and Wilkins, 1985;241–257.

11. Chievitz JH. Untersuchungen über die Verknocherung der menschlichen Kehlknorpel. Arch Anat U Entwicklungsgesch 1882:303–349.
12. Kirchner JA. Two hundred laryngeal cancers: patterns of growth and spread as seen in serial sections. Laryngoscope 1977;87:474–482.
13. Pittam MR, Carter RL. Framework invasion by laryngeal carcinomas. Head Neck Surg 1982;4:200–208.
14. Dooms GC, Hricak H, Moseley ME, Bottles K, Fisher M, Higgins CB. Characterization of lymphadenopathy by magnetic resonance relaxation times: preliminary results. Radiology 1985;155:691–697.

Chapter 8: MR imaging of normal and cancerous laryngeal cartilages. Histopathological correlation

Authors: J.A. Castelijns, M.D. (1)
G.J. Gerritsen, M.D. (2)
M.C. Kaiser, M.D. (1)
J. Valk, M.D. (1)
W. Jansen, M.D. (3)
C.J.L.M. Meyer, M.D. (3)
G.B. Snow, M.D. (2)

(1) Department of Radiology
(2) Department of Otolaryngology/
Head and Neck Surgery
(3) Department of Pathology
Institution: Free University Hospital,
Amsterdam,
The Netherlands

Abstract

MRI appearances of laryngeal cartilages, normal or invaded by cancer, are still relatively unfamiliar to the majority of clinicians. Twelve primary laryngeal tumors out of a series of 65 patients who were investigated by MRI were also examined postoperatively by macro- and microscopic sectioning of the surgical specimens. Images were obtained with a 0.6 Tesla superconductive system using a half saddle-shaped surface coil. The authors emphasize the value of a combined use of T1 weighted and proton density spin echo images. T1 weighted images permit differentiation between pathological and normal bone marrow. Proton density images allow separation between non-ossified cartilage and tumor tissue. MRI is an additional tool in the diagnostic work-up of cartilage invasion by cancer.

1. Introduction

The detection of cartilage invasion by laryngeal and hypopharyngeal carcinomas is of great clinical importance. Complications due to radiation therapy frequently occur in the presence of cartilage invasion [1]. Before the introduction of CT scanning, cartilage invasion could only very rarely be diagnosed. CT has the capacity to demonstrate gross cartilage invasion in an accurate manner, particularly when extralaryngeal tumor spread is present. However, CT fails in detecting early cartilage invasion [2]. Due to their irregular ossification laryngeal cartilages are very difficult to investigate by CT, even when a high-resolution program is used [2–5].

Uncalcified or poorly calcified cartilage may not be well displayed and erosion or destruction may thus be simulated [1–5]. On the other hand, tumor may grossly invade the medullary space of laryngeal cartilages and may not be detected if the surrounding bone is still intact [4, 6]. Earlier experience has demonstrated that by the use of specially designed surface coils it becomes possible to obtain high-signal and high-resolution magnetic resonance images of the neck with excellent soft tissue delineation [7–9]. Comparison of MR images with sliced surgical specimens showed that primary cancerous tissue was constantly seen on spin echo (SE) T1 weighted images as a homogeneous mass of intermediate signal intensity, which was slightly higher than the signal intensity of the infrahyoid muscles [10]. Gross cartilage destruction may be seen on T1 weighted images as an interruption of the cartilagineous outline [10, 11]. A comparative study of CT and MRI, utilizing a 0.15 Tesla (low field) resistive unit, has demonstrated that if bone destruction caused by head and neck lesions could be displayed CT scanning, it was equally well detected by MRI in all cases [12].

The authors studied the MRI appearances of differently ossified cartilages, invaded or uninvaded by tumor. The hyoid bone was excluded from this study because it is always ossified at an advanced age. For the present report, images generated with different SE pulse sequences (T1 weighted, proton density and T2 weighted images) were compared to corresponding macro- and microscopic slices of the surgical specimens obtained.

2. Materials and methods

Sixty five consecutive patients presenting with primary laryngeal and hypopharyngeal carcinomas at different TNM stages (according to UICC, 1978) have been investigated by MR imaging at our clinic. The patient ages ranged from 48 to 86 years. Primary carcinomas included 15 supraglottic, 38 glottic, 1 subglottic and 11 piriform sinus tumors. Recurrent diseases and residual tumors after irradiation are not included in this study. We selected the most appropriate pulse sequences and the most adequate patient and coil positioning. Images were obtained with a 0.6 Tesla superconductive system (Technicare) using a half saddle-shaped surface coil placed around the anterior aspect of the neck as a receiver antenna. An SE pulse sequence was used to obtain all images. In all three standard directions, a T1 weighted technique, which is optimal in demonstrating the anatomy, was performed using a repetition time (TR) of 200–400 ms and an echo time (TE) of 38 ms. In the axial plane we also generated at each level images using a TR of 1500 ms and a TE of 38 ms (proton density image) and 76 ms (T2 weighted image). To increase the signal-to-noise ratio the acquisition was repeated four times. The slice thickness used was 0.4 cm with a 3 mm gap. Gradient zooming was used to keep the field of view as small as possible (200 × 200 mm), so that with a 256 × 192 matrix the images had a pixel resolution of 0.8 × 1.0 mm. Acquisition times varied from 3 to 6 minutes. Twelve patients out of this group of 65 underwent laryngectomy and the specimens were obtained for organ sectioning. The surgical specimens were initially fixed in a 4% formaldehyde solution for a duration of 72 hours; then decalcification was achieved by submersion of the specimen into Kristensen's solution for approximately two weeks. According to the recommendations of Michaels and Gregor [13], axial slices with a 4 mm thickness were cut parallel to the plane of the axial MR image slices. All specimen slices were photographed and parts of the slices were processed for microscopic examination. A comparison between axial MR images, macroscopic sections and complementary microscopic findings was performed with a view to evaluate MR imaging of laryngeal cartilage, invaded or uninvaded by cancer.

3. Results

3.1. *Epiglottic cartilage*

Figures 1a and b are T1 weighted and proton density images, respectively, at the supraglottic level showing the epiglottic cartilage with intermediate signal intensity. In Fig. 1b the signal intensity is increased in comparison with Fig. 1a. On both, the thickened right ary-epiglottic fold is seen with intermediate signal intensity, which is still higher than the signal intensity of muscular tissues, but similar to that of epiglottic cartilage. This area, suspect for malignant tissue, approaches the epiglottic cartilage, but invasion of this cartilage can neither be definitely shown nor excluded. Site, contour and relation of the tumor mass to the epiglottic cartilage as seen on the T1 weighted image correspond to findings shown by the surgical specimens (Fig. 1c). Microscopically, the right portion of the epiglottic cartilage was suspect for tumor invasion (Fig. 1d).

Consequently, cancer and epiglottic cartilage can hardly be separated due to very small contrast differences on T1 weighted and proton density images.

3.2. *Thyroid cartilage*

In the next part we present two cases, in which the normal MRI appearance of thyroid cartilage is shown.

Figures 2a and b are T1 weighted and proton density axial images at the level of the false cords. Both images show segments of the thyroid cartilage with intermediate signal intensity, comparable with the signal intensity of the infrahyoid muscles. Dorsal and ventral extremes are seen with a typical three-layer appearance: a central high signal area is surrounded by rims of low signal intensity. In Fig. 2a the right paraglottic space (PGS) is infiltrated and enlarged by a homogeneous mass having an intermediate signal intensity and approaching the thyroid cartilage. Using proton density pulse sequences (Fig. 2b) this area is seen with higher signal intensity, and the contrast between thyroid cartilage and tumor tissue has increased. Macroscopic section at the corresponding level (Fig. 2c) shows tumor tissue as a white area bordering the right lamina of the thyroid cartilage. Microscopically (Fig. 2d), the right lamina is not infiltrated by tumor tissue and mainly consists of non-ossified cartilage. Its ventral and dorsal ends are ossified, showing thin trabeculae, fatty and haemopoietic tissues, surrounded by a cortical rim.

In Figs. 3a and b (T1 weighted and proton density images, respectively) the greater, i.e. ossified, part of the thyroid cartilage has a typical three-layer appearance: a central high signal area is surrounded by rims of low signal intensity. In the midportion of the left and right laminae a region of intermediate signal intensity interrupts this typical appearance. In Fig. 3a the thickened right PGS is seen with intermediate signal intensity. Invasion

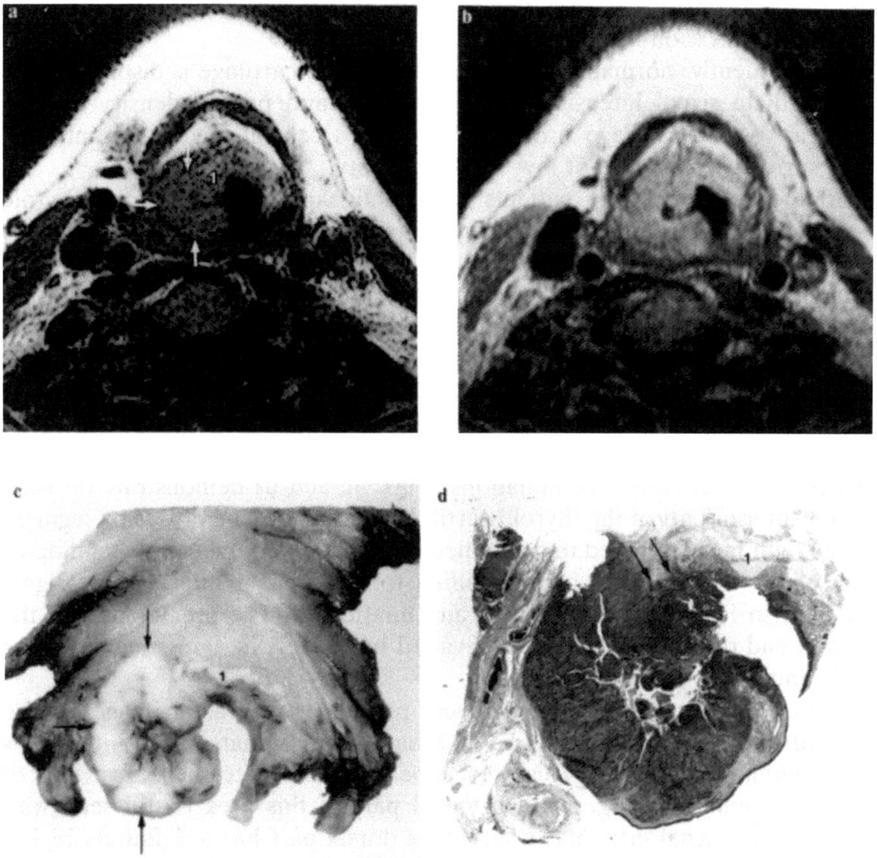

Figure 1. Case 1. Patient with T3N1 hypopharyngeal tumor.
Figure 1a. T1 weighted, axial image at a supraglottic level demonstrates tumor (arrows), contacting the epiglottic cartilage (1). Both structures are seen with similar signal intensities.
Figure 1b. On a proton density image tumor and epiglottic cartilage are both seen with increased but similar signal intensities.
Figure 1c. Sliced surgical specimen. Tumor (arrows) has similar contour and topographic relation to epiglottic cartilage (1) as shown by MRI.
Figure 1d. Microscopic section corresponding to the right posterior quadrant of the sliced specimen outlines non-ossified epiglottic cartilage (1) with tumor invasion (arrows).

of the thyroid cartilage may exist. In Fig. 3b the area which is seen in Fig. 3a within the laryngeal skeleton with intermediate signal intensity, is still seen with intermediate signal intensity, while neighbouring tissue in the PGS is seen with increased signal intensity. Corresponding macro-and microscopic (Fig. 3c and d) sections reveal that the thyroid cartilage shows advanced ossification, interrupted by areas of non-ossified cartilage within both laminae. Bone marrow consists of fat and haemapoietic tissue, lying between thin trabeculae. In this case, tumor tissue approaches the right lamina but no obvious invasion is seen.

Consequently, normal and non-ossified hyaline cartilage is displayed with intermediate signal intensity on T1 weighted and proton density images, whereas ossified cartilage is demonstrated as a central high signal intensity area surrounded by rims of low signal intensity.

In the next part, two patients with malignant invasion of the thyroid cartilage are discussed. Figures 4a and b are T1 weighted and proton density axial images just above the level of the false cords. in fig. 4a the intralaryngeal geal area is almost entirely filled by an area of intermediate signal intensity. This area extends into the prelaryngeal region, involving the infrahyoid muscles. The posterior portions of both laminae appear to be ossified. Figure 4b shows that most of the intermediate signal area of Fig. 4a has increased signal intensity, which is compatible with tumor tissue. A small region of intermediate signal intensity can still be recognized within the right lamina. Macro- and microscopic examinations (Figs. 4c and d) demonstrate invasion of the anterior part of the thyroid cartilage by cancer. The posterior segment of the right lamina proved to be ossified and unaffected, whereas the midportion of the right lamina, corresponding to the area of intermediate signal intensity in Fig. 4b, is non-ossified and unaffected. The greater part of the ventral end of the right lamina is invaded by cancer, in agreement with the MRI findings.

Figures 5a and b are T1 weighted and proton density axial images at the level of the false cords. In Fig. 5a an area of intermediate signal intensity is seen, extending laterally. This area appears to infiltrate the dorsal part of the right lamina. In Fig. 5b the ventral part of this area is still seen with intermediate signal intensity, whereas its dorsal part has a definitely higher signal intensity. Macro- and microscopic (Figs. 5c and d) sections at the corresponding level demonstrate that the tumor is entirely located within the region of intermediate signal intensity seen in Fig. 5a. The ossified and abnormal posterior portion of the right thyroid lamina (Figs. 5c and d) corresponds to the area of cartilage having increased signal intensity (Fig. 5b). Bone marrow is replaced by cancer with fibrous and inflammatory

Figure 2. Case 2. Patient with T3N0 supraglottic lesion.

Figure 2a. T1 weighted, axial image at the level of the false cords displays tumor (arrowheads) bordering the thyroid cartilage (1), which has, almost entirely, intermediate signal intensity. The ventral and dorsal ends of the right thyroid lamina are ossified (arrows).

Figure 2b. Proton density image still shows non-ossified thyroid cartilage with intermediate signal intensity. Due to increased signal intensity of cancer, contrast between tumor (arrowheads) and non-ossified cartilage has been enhanced.

Figure 2c. Macroscopic section demonstrates similar relation between tumor (arrowheads) and thyroid cartilage (1).

Figure 2d. Microscopic study of the right thyroid lamina reveals almost entirely non-ossified cartilage (1). The ventral and dorsal ends consist of bone surrounding bone marrow (arrows).

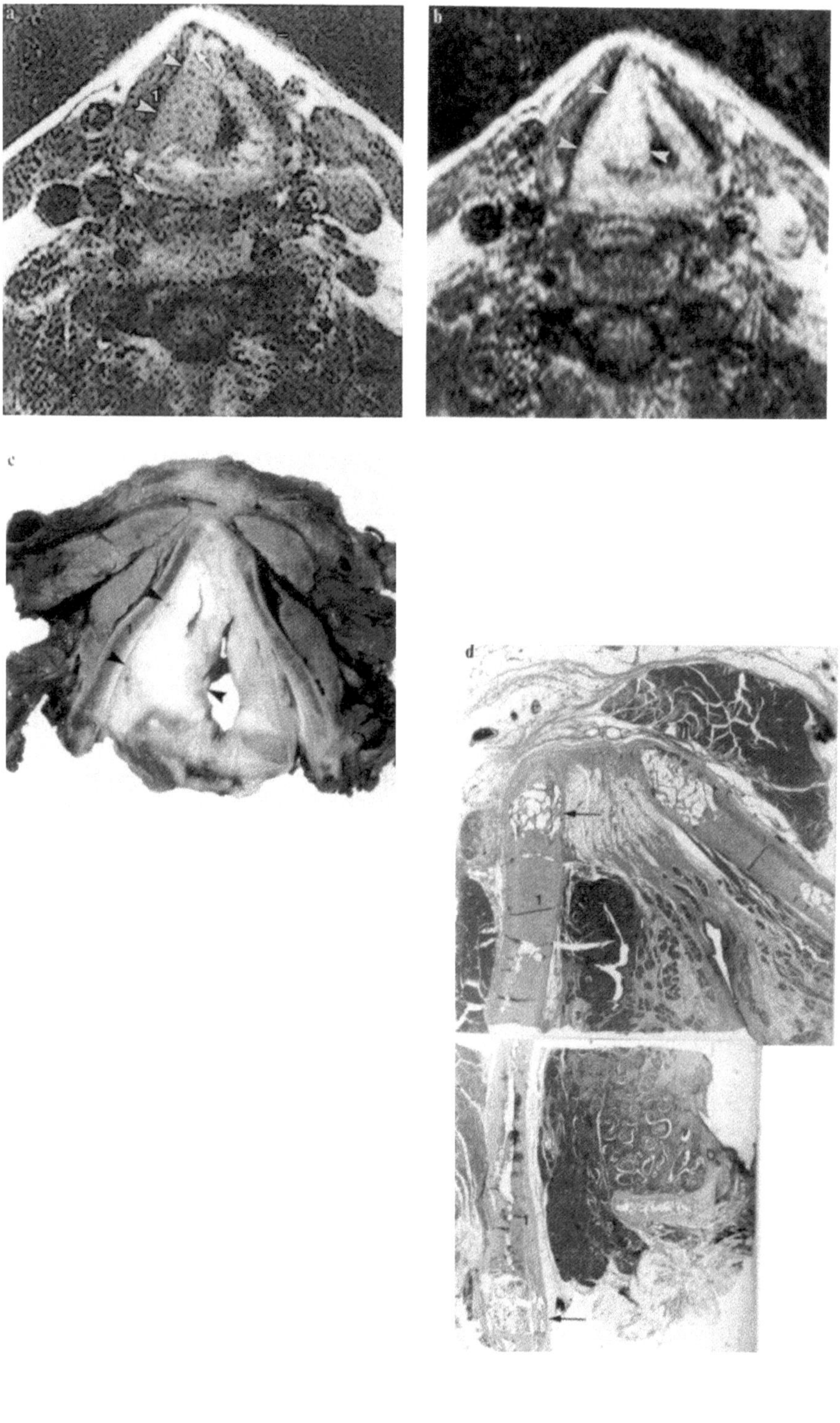
a
b
c
d

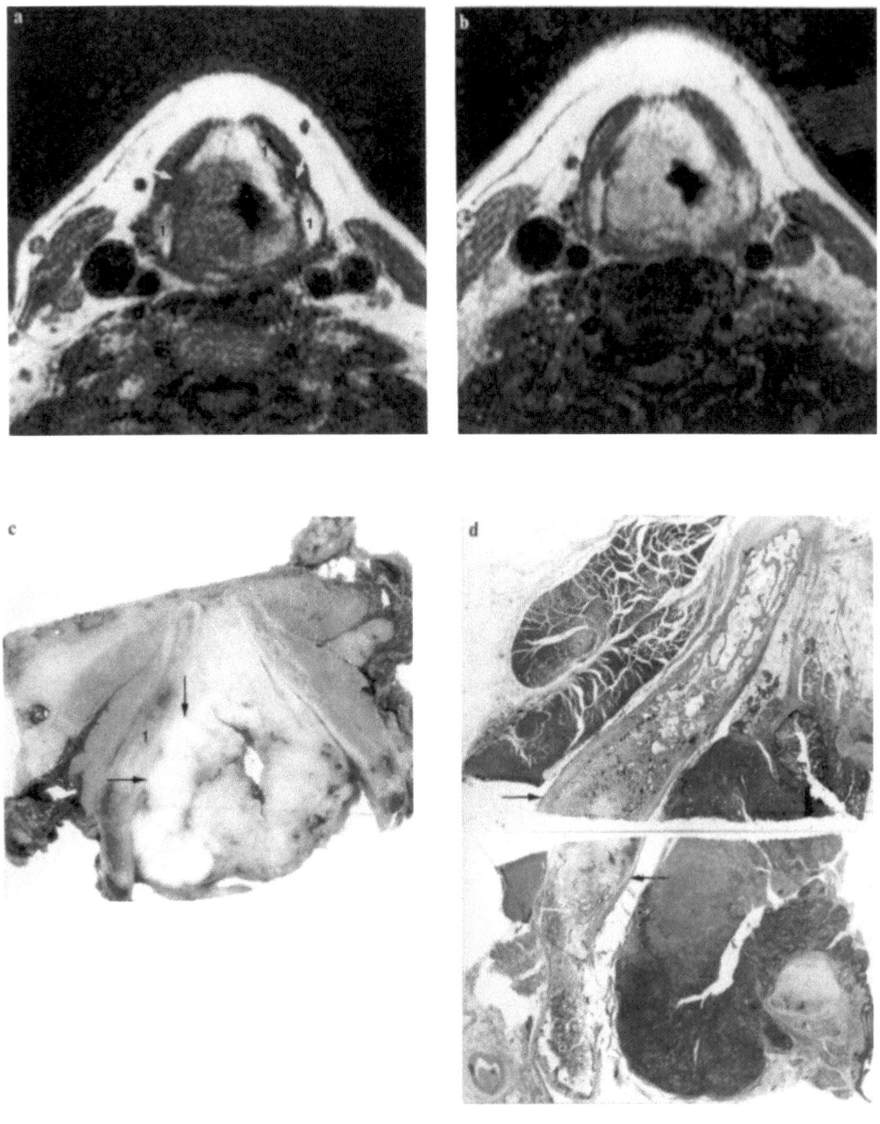

Figure 3. Case 1. Patient with T3N1 hypopharyngeal tumor.
Figure 3a. T1 weighted, axial image at the level of the false cords displays thyroid cartilage (1) which is almost entirely ossified. In the midportion of each lamina a small area of intermediate signal intensity (arrows) is seen.
Figure 3b. Proton density image still displays these areas with intermediate signal intensity.
Figure 3c. Corresponding sliced surgical specimen shows similar topographic relation of right lamina (1) to tumor (arrows), as seen on MRI examinations.
Figure 3d. Microscopic examination proves that intermediate signal intensity area of both MR images corresponds with a non-ossified portion (arrows) of the thyroid cartilage, not invaded by tumor. The remaining part of the lamina is ossified.

changes. Anteriorly, a small segment of normal, non-ossified cartilage borders the invaded region (Figs. 5c and d), which corresponds to the area of intermediate signal intensity shown in Fig. 5b. In the same patient an obvious asymmetry between the right and left thyroid laminae is also found at the level of the true vocal cords: the tumor has destroyed the dorsal portion of the right thyroid lamina (Figs. 6a and b). Pathological tissue is shown with increased signal intensity in Fig. 6b (proton density image), enhancing contrast between bone and surrounding pathological tissue. Histopathological examination (Figs. 6c and d) reveals that cancer has destroyed cartilage, the bony trabeculae being disseminated amid malignant tissue.

Consequently, malignant invasion of the thyroid cartilage is seen on the T1 weighted image with intermediate signal intensity, whereas on the proton density image it is seen with increased signal intensity.

3.3. *Cricoid cartilage*

In Figs. 7a and b (T1 and proton density images) the cricoid is seen as a central high signal area surrounded by a low intensity rim. In this case a small edge on the posterior wall of the cricoid has a lower signal intensity. On both sides, the inferior cornu of the thyroid cartilage is clearly visible lateral to the cricoid. Macro- and microscopic examinations at about the same level (Figs. 7c and d) demonstrate that the cricoid cartilage is almost entirely ossified, and is composed of fat, haemopoietic tissue and bony trabeculae. Dorsally, the cricoid is not ossified; this correlates with the MRI findings.

Figure 8a (T1 weighted) shows that the cricoid lamina is completely ossified, only a small interruption due to a mass of intermediate signal intensity is found in its right portion. This defect within the cricoid shows increased signal intensity in Figure 8b (proton density image), which raises the suspicion of cartilage invasion. Macro- and microscopic examinations (Figs. 8c and d) confirm tumor infiltration into the ossified cricoid. In regard to the tumor site and contour, a striking correlation was found between pathologic findings and MR images. Histopathologic examination (Fig. 8d) demonstrates cancer invading the ossified cricoid.

Gross invasion of cartilagineous structures is seen in Figs. 9a and b: the right inferior cornu of the thyroid cartilage and the greater part of the cricoid lamina are imaged with intermediate (Fig. 9a) and increased (Fig. 9b) signal intensity. This finding is suggestive of massive invasion by cancer. MRI findings were confirmed by examination of the surgical specimens (Figs. 9c and d). Thus, signal intensities of normal and invaded cricoid cartilages as shown by MRI are similar to those of normal and invaded thyroid cartilages.

3.4. *Arytenoid cartilage*

Figures 6a and b show ossification of both arytenoids. In Fig. 6a (T1 weighted) an area with homogeneous intermediate signal intensity, suspect for cancer, borders on the right arytenoid. No evidence of invasion is seen. Slices of the surgical specimens at the corresponding level (Figs. 6c and d) show almost complete ossification of the arytenoids. Their vocal processes are still cartilagineous. Cancer borders on the right arytenoid, but no signs of invasion are seen.

4. Discussion

The signal intensity of tissues as imaged by MRI is predominantly dependent upon the proton density and the highly heterogeneous distribution of the T1 and T2 spin-relaxation rates in the various tissues. Protons raising MRI signals are mainly located in tissue water and lipids. Protons in solid structures (e.g. bone) do not contribute to the signal. Tissue contrast may be manipulated by choosing variable pulse sequences (TE, TR), accentuating the effects of differences in T1 or T2 spin-relaxation rates. As a rule, tumor tissue is imaged with intermediate signal intensity on T1 weighted images, whereas on more T2 weighted images its signal intensity increases [14, 15]. Primary laryngeal cancer is constantly seen on T1 weighted images as a homogeneous mass of intermediate signal intensity, which in all cases is slightly higher than the signal intensity of the infrahyoid muscles. Site, extension and contour of the tumor mass, as shown by axial MRI examinations, corresponds to the actual configuration of the lesion [10]. T2 weighted images, obtained by using a long TR (1500 ms) and TE (76 ms), have a low signal-to-noise ratio (not shown), in agreement with the findings of Lufkin et al. [11]. Using a long TR (1500 ms) and a short TE (38 ms), T1 as well as T2 tissue characteristics are accentuated on the images obtained. In our opinion, this technique is a good compromise between a reasonable signal-to-noise ratio and an adequate expression of T2 values, because tumor tissue is still seen with increased signal intensity.

Figure 4. Case 3. Patient with T4N0 transglottic lesion.
Figure 4a. T1 weighted, axial image at the level of the ary-epiglottic folds shows tumor (arrows), invading the thyroid cartilage (1) and infiltrating the infrahyoid muscles (2).
Figure 4b. Proton density image. A small area of intermediate signal intensity (arrow) separates the invaded ventral extreme and the normal ossified dorsal extreme of the right thyroid lamina.
Figure 4c. Sliced specimen demonstrates tumor (arrows) with a similar topographic relation to thyroid cartilage (1) and infrahyoid muscles (2), as demonstrated by MRI.
Figure 4d. Microscopy shows, that the area of intermediate signal intensity on Figure 4b consists of non-ossified cartilage (arrows), whereas the ventral part of the thyroid lamina (1) is invaded by cancer.

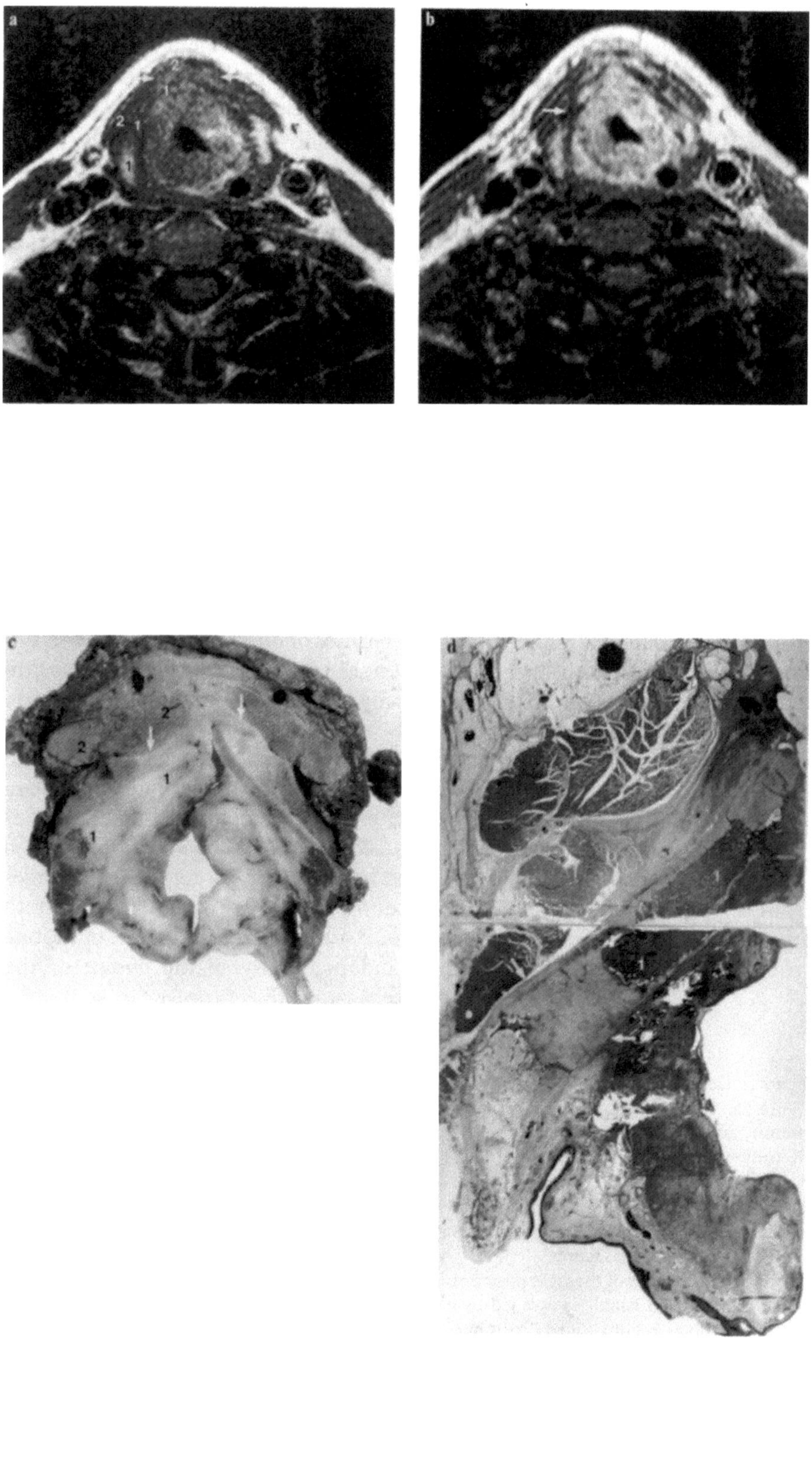
a
b
c
d

The epiglottic cartilage and the vocal processes of the arytenoids are composed of yellow fibrocartilage, which usually does not ossify. The T1 weighted image (Fig. 1a) demonstrates the epiglottic cartilage with intermediate signal intensity. On the proton density image (Fig. 1b) it is seen with increased signal intensity compared to T1 weighted images. On both types of images the contrast between tumor and cartilage is minimal. Although the vicinity of a tumor to the epiglottic cartilage may be cause for suspicion of invasion, invasion of the epiglottic cartilage may neither be definitely demonstrated nor excluded by MRI. This finding agrees with earlier experience [10]. The cricoid, thyroid and the greater part of the arytenoid consist of hyaline cartilage. These hyaline cartilages begin their ossification between the ages of 20 and 25 years. Keen and Wainwright concluded that the microscopic changes essentially consist of normal endochondral ossification [16]. It remains impossible to formulate precise laws about the macroscopic pattern of this ossification, as there is a high degree of variability between individuals. Furthermore, in relation to age, ossification proceeds in a very irregular way [17]. At an age when cancer is likely to occur, cartilages consist of variable amounts of hyaline cartilage, ossified tissues and bone marrow, the latter containing fat and haemopoietic tissues lying within thin trabeculae of bone.

We turn now to a discussion of the MRI appearances of normal, non-ossified and ossified, hyaline cartilages. Non-ossified hyaline cartilage is imaged with intermediate signal intensity on T1 weighted as well as on proton density images (Figs. 2–6). Upon increasing the T2 accentuation, particularly by delaying TE, non-ossified cartilage is seen with lower intensity (not shown). Tissue contrast between non-ossified cartilage and malignant tissue is minimal on T1 weighted images (Figs. 2a, 3a), but is remarkably enhanced on proton density images as the signal intensity of malignant tissue increases strongly (Figs. 2b, 3b). Ossified cartilage is composed of compact bone which surrounds bone marrow. On T1 weighted as well as on proton density images it has a typical three-layered appearance: a central high signal area on both sides bounded by low intensity rims (Figs. 3–9). Because of its lack of mobile protons, cortical bone appears black, independently of the choice of the

Figure 5. Case 4. Patient with T4N1 hypopharyngeal tumor.

Figure 5a. T1 weighted, axial image of the level of the false cords. Large intermediate signal intensity area, suspect for tumor (arrows), extends laterally, producing intermediate signal intensity within the dorsal extreme of the right lamina (1).

Figure 5b. On the proton density image the low signal area inside the right lamina is subdivided into two regions: the ventral region (arrow) still has an intermediate signal intensity, whereas the dorsal region (arrowhead) has an increased signal intensity.

Figure 5c. Macroscopic section.

Figure 5d. Microscopy of the right posterior quadrant of Figure 5c proves that the dorsal extreme of the right thyroid lamina is invaded by cancer and reactive tissues (arrows). Ventral to this area the cartilage is not ossified (arrowheads).

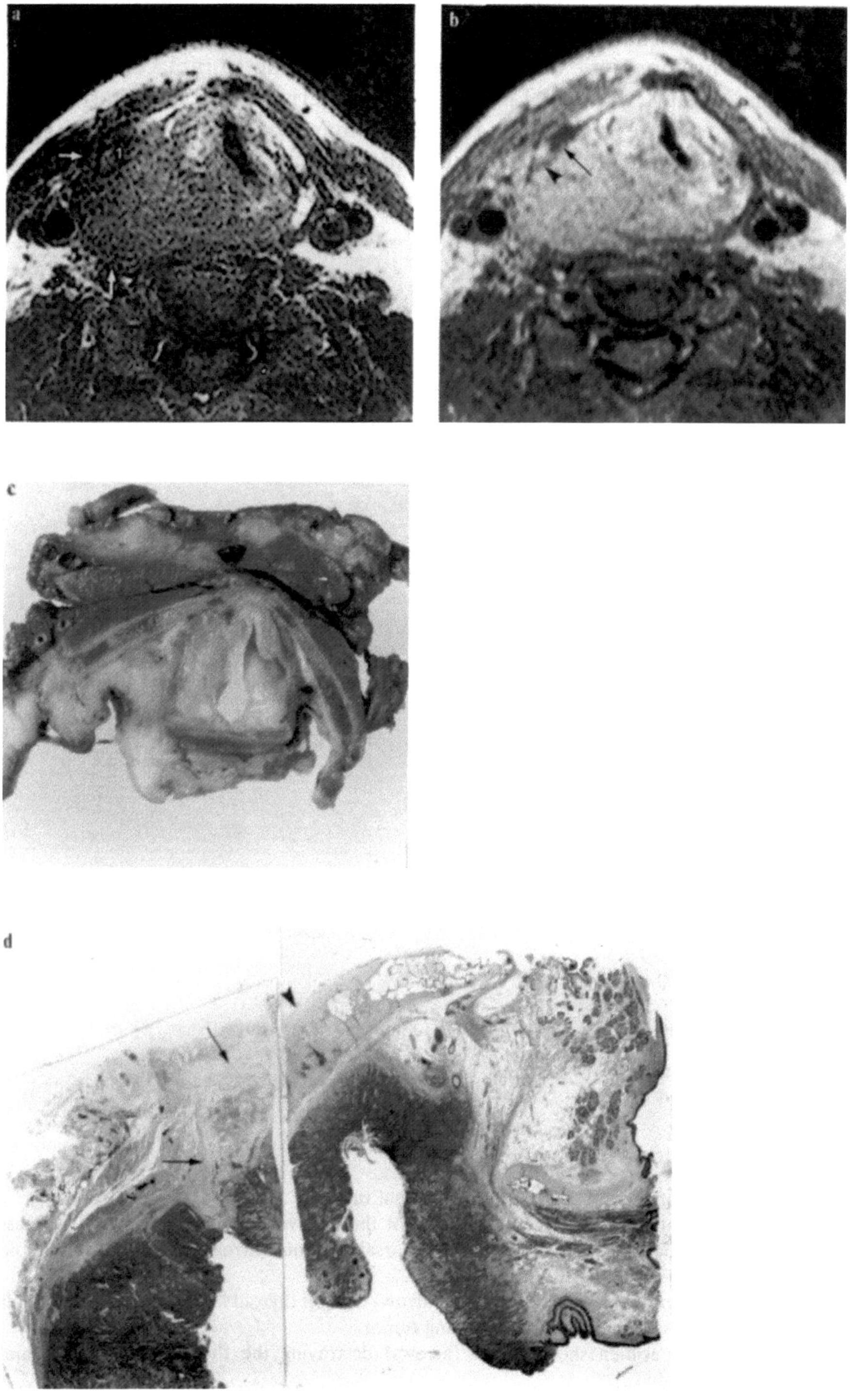
a
b
c
d

pulse sequences [15]. Bone marrow mainly consists of fatty tissue, and to a lesser degree, of haemopoietic tissue. With aging, there is a progressive decrease of haemopoietic tissues in bone marrow due to replacement by fat [18]. This explains why the T1 and T2 characteristics of bone marrow are very similar to those of fat. As a rule, bone marrow is seen with high signal intensity on T1 weighted images, much higher than the signal intensity due

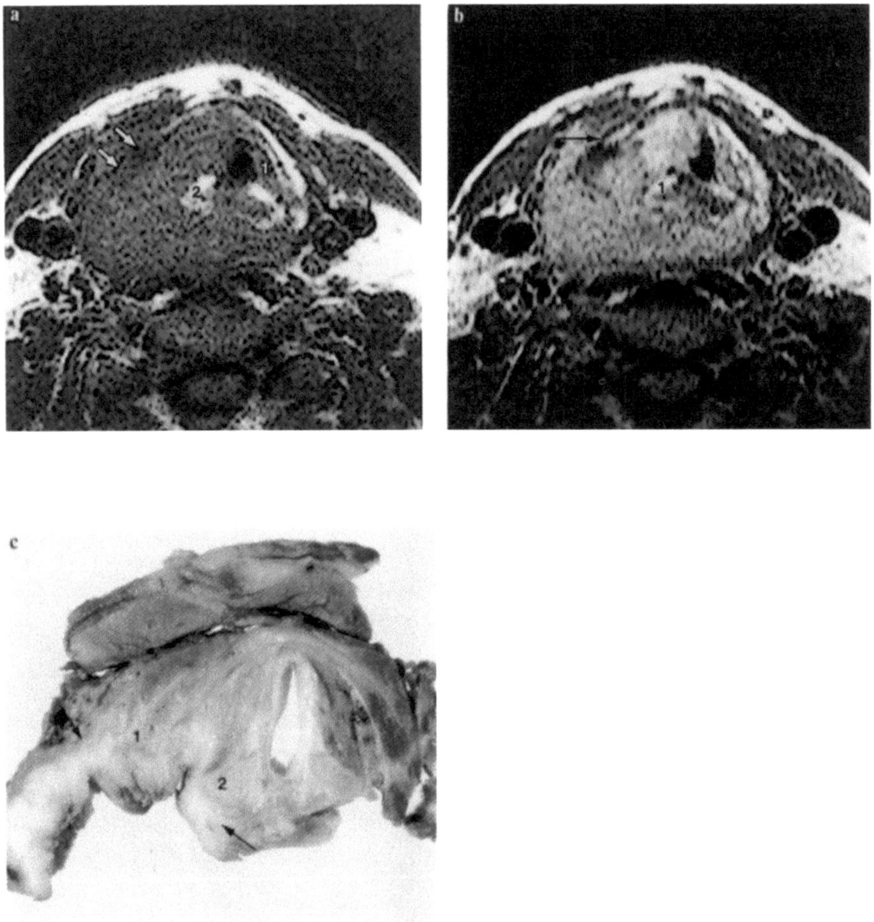

Figure 6. Case 4. Patient with T4N1 hypopharyngeal tumor.
Figure 6a. T1 weighted, axial image of the level of the true vocal cords (1) shows lårge mass of intermediate signal intensity destroying the dorsal extreme (arrows) of the right thyroid lamina, whereas the arytenoids (2) are still intact.
Figure 6b. Proton density image displays bone (arrow) of right thyroid lamina and the arytenoids (1) with high contrast compared to surrounding tumor.
Figure 6c. Sliced specimen shows tumor (arrows) destroying the thyroid cartilage (1) and touching the arytenoid (2).

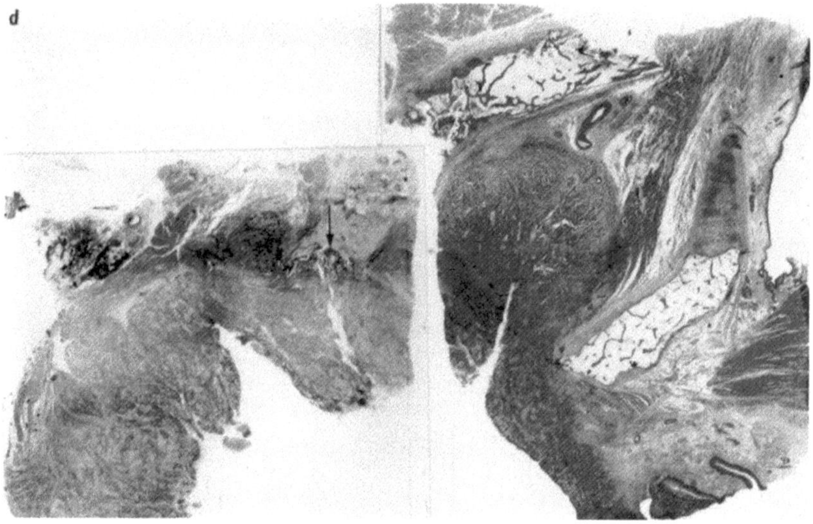

Figure 6d. Microscopy of the right half confirms cortical destruction (arrow).

to tumor. In the majority of cases in which cartilage invasion by cancer occurs, the invasion remains confined to its ossified portions [19]. On T1 weighted images cancer, invading cartilage is shown as an area of intermediate signal intensity (Figs. 4a, 6a, 8a and 9a). If the medullary space is involved, tumor is still seen with intermediate signal intensity, which is

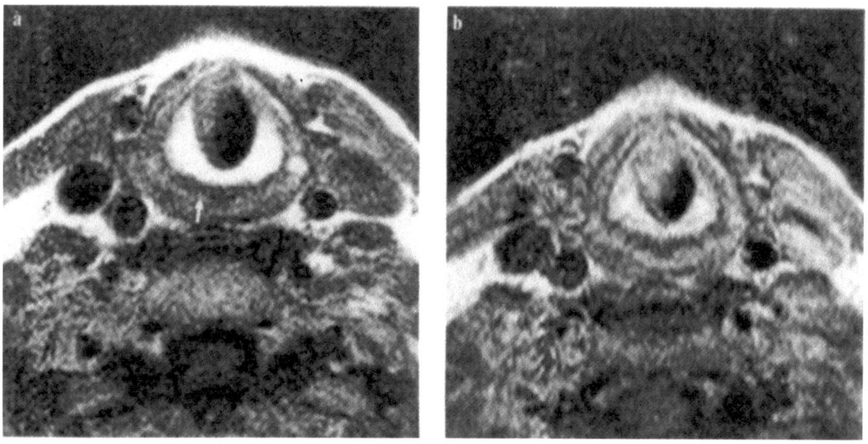

Figure 7. Case 2. Patient with T3N0 supraglottic tumor.
Figure 7a. T1 weighted, axial image at subglottic level shows that the cricoid is almost entirely ossified. Its dorsal portion (arrow) has an intermediate signal intensity.
Figure 7b. Proton density image still displays the dorsal part of the cricoid with intermediate signal intensity.

c

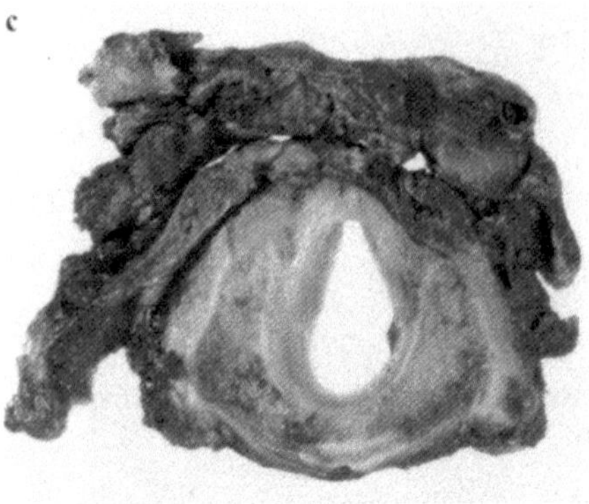

d

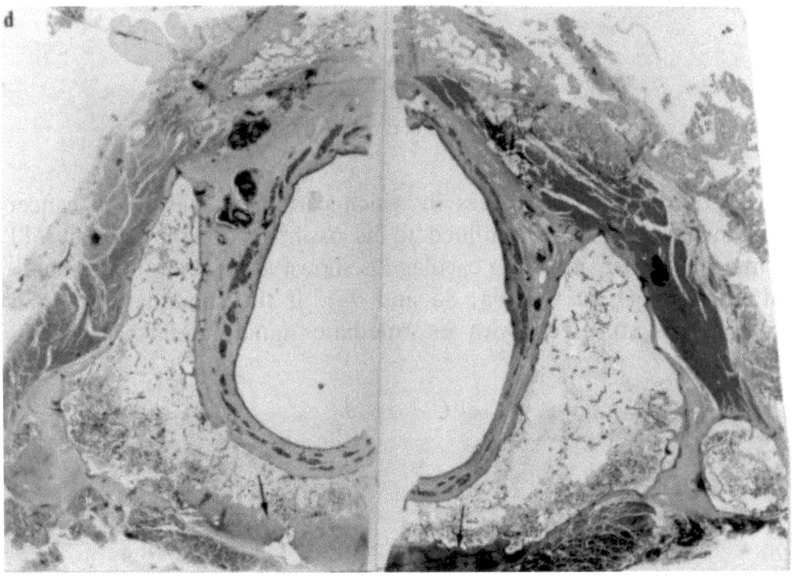

Figure 7c. Macroscopic section at about the same level.
Figure 7d. Microscopy proves that the corresponding area (arrows) of intermediate signal intensity on both MRI scans is not ossified.

different from the high signal intensity of normal bone marrow but similar to the MRI appearance of non-ossified cartilage (Figs. 4a, 6a). Since CT might not detect gross invasion of the medullary space, MRI may provide additional diagnostic information. Differentiating invaded cartilage from non-ossified cartilage is a major diagnostic challenge in order to confirm or exclude cartilage invasion. Whereas both tissues are seen on T1 weighted image with intermediate signal intensity (Figs. 4a, 6a), they are imaged with high contrast on proton density images (Figs. 4b, 6b), because tumor tissue,

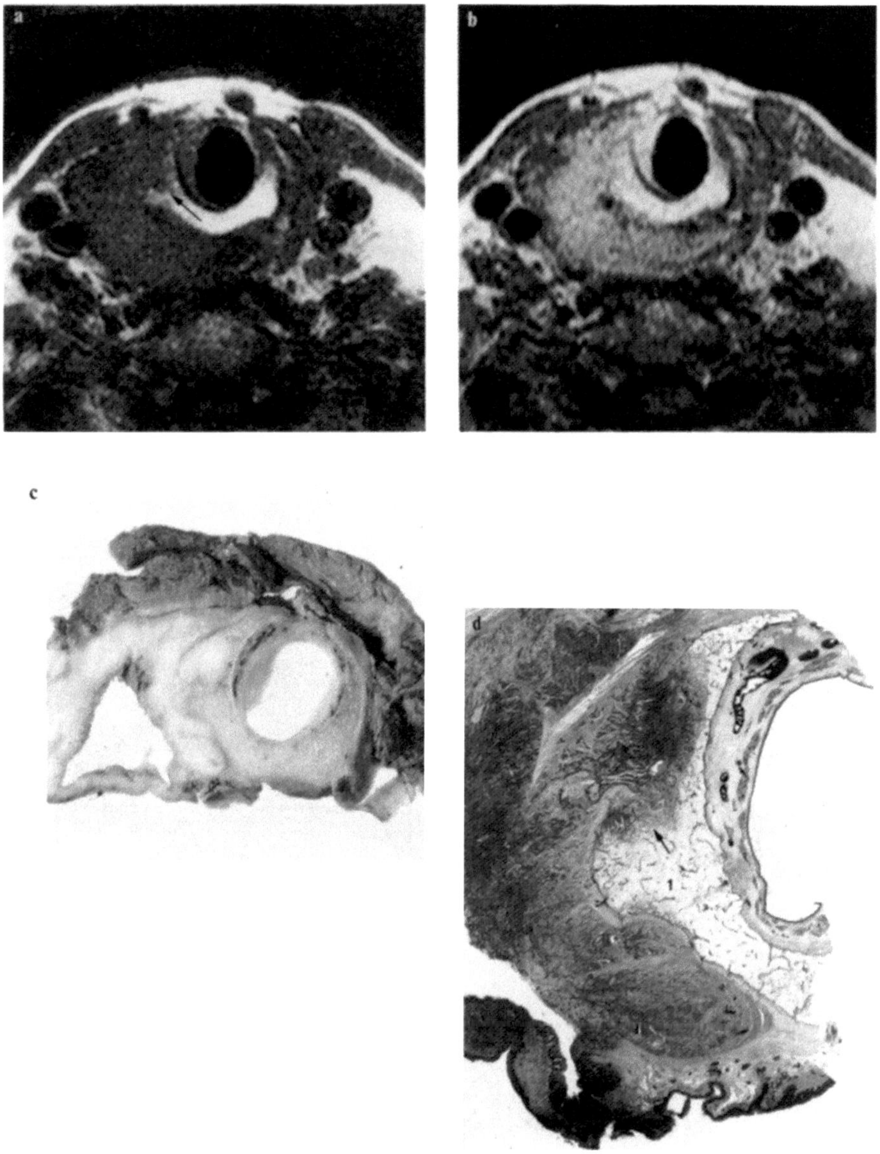

Figure 8. Case 4. Patient with T4N1 hypopharyngeal tumor.

Figure 8a. T1 weighted, axial image at the subglottic level shows minor infiltration (arrow) of the cricoid by a mass of intermediate signal intensity.

Figure 8b. Proton density image displays area, suspect for infiltration, with increased signal intensity.

Figure 8c. Sliced surgical specimen demonstrates that the right wall of the cricoid is invaded by tumor.

Figure 8d. Microscopic section of the right half demonstrates cancer infiltrating the cricoid (arrows).

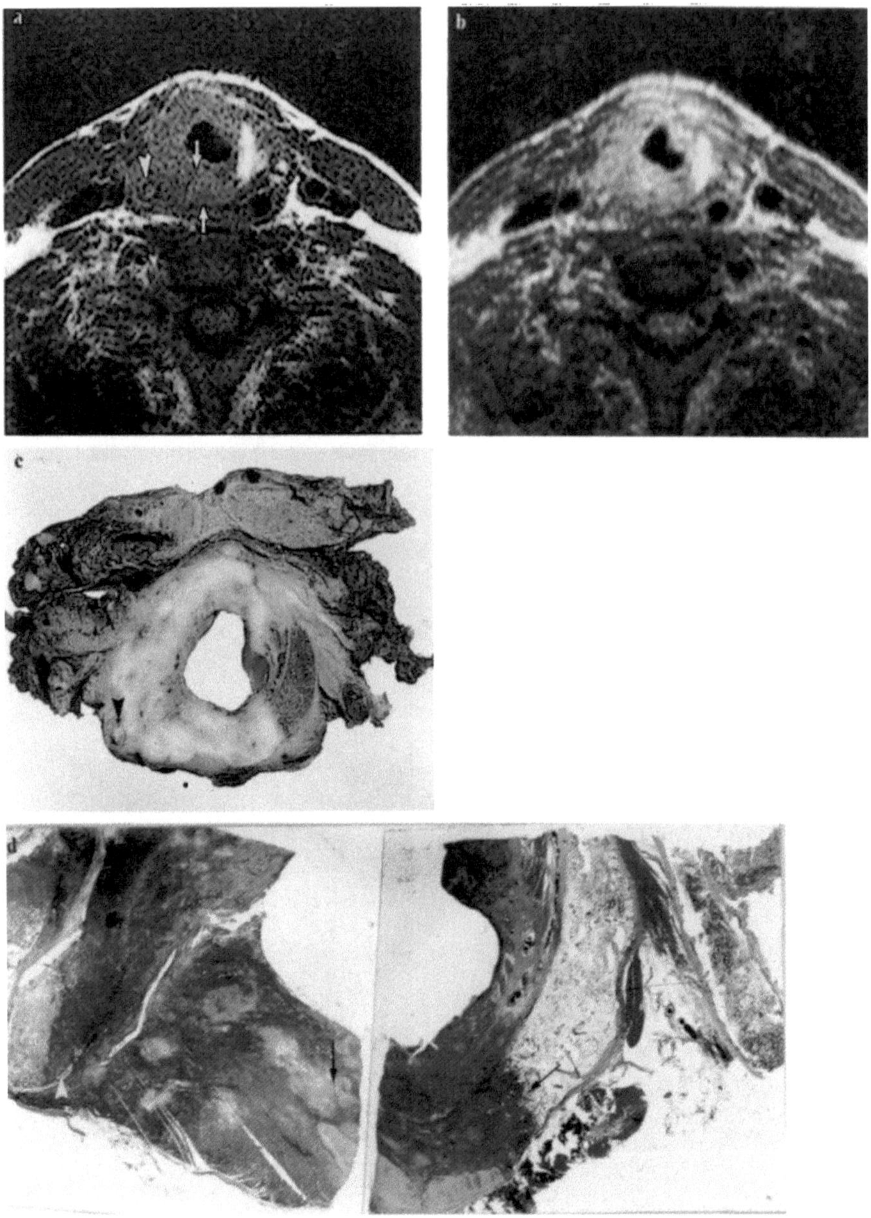

Figure 9. Case 3. Patient with T4N0 transglottic tumor.
Figure 9a. T1 weighted, axial image at subglottic level shows large tumorous area invading the right inferior cornu of the thyroid cartilage (arrowheads) and the greater part (arrows) of the cricoid.
Figure 9b. Proton density image displays tumor with increased signal intensity.
Figure 9c. A similar contour of the tumor, invading both the right inferior cornu (arrowheads) and the cricoid, is macroscopically seen.
Figure 9d. Microscopic section shows cancer infiltrating the cricoid (arrows) and the right inferior cornu (arrowhead) of the thyroid cartilage.

Table 1. Relative signal intensities of different tissue types on T1 weighted and proton density images.

	T1–weighted	Proton density
Elastic cartilage	Intermediate	Intermediate
Hyaline cartilage	Intermediate	Intermediate
Compact bone	Low	Low
Bone marrow (fatty-, haemapoietic)	High	High
Cancer (invading and non-invading	Intermediate	Intermediate to high

invading and non-invading, is found to have an increased signal intensity and non-ossified cartilage still has an intermediate signal intensity (Figs. 2–7).

5. Conclusions

Gross cartilage invasion is clearly demonstrated by MRI. In order to be able to diagnose minor invasion of hyaline cartilages the combined use of SE T1 weighted and proton density images can be very helpful (Figs. 4, 8). In our experience it is possible to distinguish affected cartilage from normal bone marrow by the use of T1 weighted images on the one hand, and from non-ossified cartilage by the use of proton density images on the other hand (Table 1). Comparative assessment of MRI and CT results should ascertain the value of this statement.

References

1. Gerritsen GJ, Valk J, van Velzen DJ, Snow GB. Computed Tomography: a mandatory investigational procedure for the T-staging of advanced laryngeal cancer. Clin Otolaryngol 1986;11:307–316.
2. Mafee MF, Schild JA, Michael AS, Choi KH, Capek V. Cartilage involvement in laryngeal carcinoma: correlation of CT and pathologic macrosection studies. J Comput Assist Tomogr 1985;8(5):969–73.
3. Hoover LA, Calcaterra TC, Waler GA, Larrson SG. Preoperative CT scan evaluation for laryngeal carcinoma: correlation with pathological findings. Laryngoscope 1984;94:310–315.
4. Silverman PM, Bossen EH, Fisher SR, Boyce Cole T, Korobkin L, Halvorsen RA. Carcinoma of the Larynx and Hypopharynx: Computed Tomographic-histopathologic Correlations. Radiology 1984;151:697–702.
5. Yeager VL, Lawson C, Archer CR. Ossification of the laryngeal cartilages as it relates to computed tomography. Invest Radiol 1982;17:11–19.
6. Archer CR, Yeager VL. Computed tomography of laryngeal cancer with histopathological correlation. Laryngoscope 1982;92:1173–1180.
7. McArdle CB, Bailey BJ, Amparo EG. Surface coil magnetic resonance imaging of the normal larynx. Arch Otolaryngol Head and Neck Surg 1986;112:616–622.
8. Castelijns JA, Doornbos J, Verbeeten B Jr, Vielvoye GJ, Bloem JL. Magnetic Resonance Imaging 1985;9(5):919–25.

9. Lufkin RB, Hanafee WN. Application of surface coils to MR anatomy of the larynx. AJNR 1985;6:491–497.
10. Castelijns JA, Kaiser MC, Valk J, Gerritsen GJ, van Hattum AH, Snow GB. MRI of laryngeal cancer. J Comput Assist Tomogr 1987;11(1):134–140.
11. Lufkin RB, Hanafee WN, Wortham D, Hoover L. Larynx and hypopharynx: MR imaging with surface coils. Radiology 1986;158:747–754.
12. Vriapangse C, Mancuso A, Fitzsimmons J, Gainsville. Value of magnetic resonance imaging in assessing one destruction in head in neck lesions. Laryngoscope 1986;96:284–291.
13. Michaels L, Gregor RT. Examination of the larynx in the histopathology laboratory. J Clin Pathol 1980;33:705–709.
14. Valk J, MacLean C, Algra PR. The clinical application of NMR tomography. In: Valk J ed. Basic principles of nuclear magnetic resonance imaging. Amsterdam-New York-Oxford, Elsevier 1985:115–140.
15. Wehrli FW, MacFalk JR, Newton TH. Parameters determining the appearance of NMR images. In: advanced imaging techniques. Modern neuroradiology, Vol.2. Newton TH, Potts DG, Eds. Clavandel Press, San Anselmo 1983:81–117.
16. Keen JA, Wainwright JS. Ossification of the thyroid, cricoid and arytenoid cartilages. S Afr J Lab Clin Med 1958:4:83–108.
17. Roncallo P. Researches about ossification and conformation of the thyroid cartilage in men. Acta Otolaryng 1948;36:110–134.
18. Dooms GC, Fisher, MR, Hricak H, Richardson M, Crooks LE, Genant HK. Bone marrow imaging: magnetic resonance studies related to age and sex. Radiology 1985;155:429–432.
19. Kirchner JA. Two hundred laryngeal cancers: patterns of growth and spread as seen in serial Sections. The Laryngoscope 1977;87:474–480.

Chapter 9: Diagnosis of laryngeal cartilage invasion by cancer. Comparison of CT and MR imaging

Authors: J.A. Castelijns, M.D. (1)
G.J. Gerritsen, M.D. (2)
M.C. Kaiser, M.D. (1)
J. Valk, M.D. (1)
T.E.G. van Zanten , M.D. (1)
R.G. Golding, F.R.C.P. (1)
C.J.L.M. Meyer, M.D. (3)
A.H. van Hattum, M.D. (3)
M. Sprenger, Ph.D. (4)
P.D. Bezemer, Ph.D. (5)
G.B. Snow, M.D. (2)

(1) Department of Radiology
(2) Department of Otolaryngology/Head and Neck Surgery
(3) Department of Pathology
(4) Instruments Department
(5) Medical Statistics

Institution: Free University Hospital
Amsterdam
The Netherlands

-

Abstract

Forty-two patients with laryngeal carcinomas were examined by Computed Tomography (CT) and Magnetic Resonance Imaging (MRI). The accuracy of CT and MRI in showing cartilage invasion was evaluated in 16 patients by comparing the results with pathological findings. Calcified cartilage, invaded by cancer, is frequently seen with CT as having an intact contour, whereas tumor approaching non-ossified cartilage may simulate cartilage invasion. On the other hand, T1 weighted MR images demonstrate invaded bone marrow of ossified cartilage with intermediate signal intensity, which allows its differentiation from normal bone marrow. Proton density images show tumor with increased signal intensity, which permits one to differentiate the latter from non-ossified cartilage. In our experience, the specificities of CT and MRI were approximately equal, 91 and 88%, respectively. CT has a definitely lower sensitivity than MRI (46 and 89%, respectively). Gross movement artifacts, which resulted in non-diagnostic images, occurred in 16% of the MRI examinations.

We recommend MRI as the modality of choice in the diagnosis of cartilage invasion.

1. Introduction

The introduction of computed tomography (CT) has contributed significantly to the study of larynx and hypopharynx. The important value of CT in the diagnostic evaluation of laryngeal cancer was found in its ability to display submucous extension of tumor and, in particular, gross cartilage invasion [1]. However, CT failed in detecting minor cartilage invasion, due to extreme variations in calcifications [2, 3]. In a recent publication on advanced laryngeal cancer, unrecognized cartilage invasion occurred with a frequency of 25% [4]. Compared to CT, Magnetic Resonance (MR) imaging, with its improved soft tissue contrast and its ability to perform multiplanar imaging, is an appealing modality for the study of head and neck pathology. The use of specially designed surface coils has provided the possibility to obtain high-signal and high-resolution MR images of the neck with excellent soft tissue delineation [5–8]. A previous study showed that patients suffering from dyspnea could successfully be imaged diagnostically by using shorter examination times with an appropriate choice of pulse parameters, acquisition matr-

Table 1. Relative signal intensities of various tissue types

Tissue type	Signal intensity T1 weighted image	Proton density image
Hyaline cartilage	Intermediate	Intermediate
Compact bone	Low	Low
Bone marrow	High	High
Cancer	Intermediate	Intermediate to high

ices and a minimum number of slices [14]. In our hands MR examinations failed in patients with recurrent tumor after irradiation treatment, because distinction between residual or recurrent tumor, radiation fibrosis and edema was not possible [14]. In a previous report it was stated that the combined use of T1 weighted and proton density images in the axial plane allows MRI to be is a promising additional tool in the diagnostic work-up of cartilage invasion in patients who have not been previously treated. T1 weighted axial images permit differentiation between pathological and normal bone marrow. Proton density axial images allow separation between non-ossified cartilage and tumor tissue [9, 10] (Table 1).

In the present study we have compared the CT and MRI appearances of laryngeal cartilage invasion by cancer in previously untreated patients by using macro- and microscopic specimens as a standard of reference. In addition, we have evaluated the diagnostic accuracy of MRI and CT in the diagnosis of cartilage invasion by comparing findings of multiple observers with histopathologic observations.

2. Materials and methods

Forty two patients with clinically proven and previously untreated laryngeal or hypopharyngeal cancer were examined by MRI and CT. Sixteen patients underwent surgery. Twenty six patients were treated with irradiation treatment. There were 38 (15) men and 4 (1) woman with ages ranging between 46 (52) and 87 (76) years. The number of patients who underwent surgery are reported between brackets. Primary carcinomas included 17 (4) supraglottic, 16 (8) (trans)glottic, 1 (0) subglottic and 8 (4) hypopharyngeal tumors. All patients had a squamous cell carcinoma.

The CT scans were obtained within two weeks before and after the MRI study: 22 scans were obtained before MRI, and 20 CT scans after MR examinations. MRI and CT were performed independently. To avoid bias caused by patient selection, our MR series was a consecutive one, although patients carrying a pacemaker, or who were in poor clinical condition, had to be excluded from this study. At our institution, all patients with supraglottic tumor and patients with an advanced glottic or subglottic tumor, clinically staged as T3 and T4, routinely undergo CT examination.

2.1. *Imaging techniques*

CT scanning was performed using a third generation scanner, (Philips Tomoscan 350). The slice thickness used were 3, 4.5 or 6 mm with no interslice gap. The field of view was 240 × 240 mm. The scanning time was 9 seconds. Patients were asked to breathe normally. MR images were obtained on a 0.6 Tesla superconductive system (Technicare-Tescalon I) using a half saddle-shaped surface coil placed around the anterior aspect of the neck. A multisection two-dimensional Fourier transform spin-echo (SE) pulse sequence was used in all cases. In sagittal, axial and frontal planes T1 weighted images were obtained using a repetition time (TR) of 200–400 ms and an echo time (TE) of 38 ms. In the axial plane we also generated proton density (SE 1500/38) and T2 weighted (SE 1500/76) images at each corresponding level. The acquisition of T1 weighted images was repeated four times for signal averaging, whereas the acquisition of proton density images and T2 weighted images was repeated twice. The slice thickness used was 4 mm with a 3 mm interslice gap. The field of view was kept as small as possible (200 × 200 mm) so that, with a 256 × 192 acquisition matrix, the T1 weighted images had a pixel resolution of 0.8 × 1.0 mm. Proton density and T2 weighted images had a 256 × 128 acquisition matrix. Acquisition times varied from 3 to 6 minutes. Patients were instructed to breathe quietly and to refrain from swallowing.

2.2. *Image interpretation*

All CT and MRI studies were retrospectively reviewed by two pairs of two independent observers, who were asked to assess the presence of cartilage invasion. Observers of CT scans (T.v.Z., R.G.) were familiar with the evaluation of CT examinations of the larynx. MRI observers (M.K., J.V.) were trained in evaluating MRI examinations. The observers were "blind" to the results of the other study, to previous interpretations of the studies, and to clinical information and therapeutic decisions. At the end of the first set of readings, the reviewers of each modality compared their findings. In cases of disagreement, both readers of each modality reviewed the examinations together to reach a consensus. The radiological and pathological findings are tabulated in Table 2. There were 16 cases of disagreement (one observer diagnosed "probably" or "evident" cartilage invasion and the other one diagnosed "probably no" or "no" invasion) between CT observers and 18 cases of disagreement between MRI observers. In order to evaluate movement artifacts, all observers were asked whether adequate interpretation of images was possible.

Table 2. Cartilage findings in surgically treated patients

		Cartilage Findings														
		Epiglottic			Thyroid			Left Arytenoid			Right Arytenoid			Cricoid		
Patient	Tumor Site/Stage	CT	MR	HP	CT	MR	HP	CT	MR	HP	CT	MR	HP	CT	MR	HP
1	Supraglottic/T1b	--	+	++	--	+	++	--	-	--	--	--	--	--	--	--
2	Glottic/T3	--	-	--	++	++	++	-	+	++	--	--	--	++	++	++
3	Supraglottic/T3	--	--	--	-	+	++	--	--	--	--	-	--	--	--	--
4	Glottic/T3	--	+	++	-	+	++	--	--	--	--	-	--	--	--	--
5	Glottic/T3	-	++	++	++	++	++	+	-	--	-	++	++	-	++	++
6	Glottic/T3	-	++	++	+	-	++	--	--	--	-	-	++	--	--	--
7	Glottic/T3	++	++	++	++	++	++	+	++	++	--	-	--	++	+	--
8	Glottic/T3	+	++	++	++	++	++	--	+	--	-	++	++	-	++	++
9	Glottic/T3	--	++	++	+	++	++	--	+	++	--	-	--	--	+	++
10	Supraglottic/T4	+	+	++	--	--	--	--	--	--	--	--	--	--	--	--
11	Supraglottic/T1b	+	+	++	--	--	--	--	--	--	--	--	--	--	--	--
12	Glottic/T3	--	+	++	--	+	++	--	+	++	--	--	--	--	-	--
13	Hypopharyngeal/T3	+	+	++	+	++	--	--	--	--	--	++	--	--	-	--
14	Hypopharyngeal/T3	+	-	++	+	+	++	--	-	--	++	+	--	-	--	--
15	Hypopharyngeal/T4	-	-	--	++	++	++	--	--	--	++	-	++	--	++	++
16	Hypopharyngeal/T2	--	--	--	--	--	--	-	--	--	--	--	--	--	--	--

Note.—HP = histopathologic findings; ++ = invasion evident; + = invasion probable; - = invasion unlikely; -- = no invasion

2.3. *Pathological findings*

Thirteen patients underwent total laryngectomy and three patients underwent supraglottic laryngectomy (15 patients within one month after using both examinations). Since the margin of resection of three supraglottic specimens was free of tumor, we concluded that the arytenoids and the cricoid were not invaded in these patients. The surgical specimens were obtained for organ sectioning. They were initially fixed for a period of 72 hours in a 4% formaldehyde solution; then decalcified by submersion of the specimen into Kristensen's solution for approximately two weeks. According to the recommendations of Michaels and Gregor [11], axial 4 mm thick slices were cut parallel to the plane of the axial CT and MR images. Parts of all the slices were processed for microscopic examination.

3. Results

3.1. *Epiglottic cartilage*

An axial CT scan (Fig. 1a) at the supraglottic level of a male patient (No. 16) with a hypopharyngeal lesion, clinically staged as T2N1, shows the left piriform sinus filled with a tumor mass. Tumor, which is seen with increased density, does not extend to the region of the epiglottic cartilage. Therefore invasion of this cartilage may be excluded. The patient also underwent MR examination. In Fig. 1b, which is a T1 weighted image, the same area is seen with intermediate signal intensity, suggestive of cancer. Because the epiglottic cartilage is surrounded by tissue having the normally high signal intensity of fat, invasion of the epiglottic cartilage may be excluded. Microscopy confirmed the MRI findings (Fig. 1d).

An axial CT scan (Fig. 2a), just above the level of the false cords in a male patient (No. 4) with a T3NO transglottic lesion, shows thickening within the dorsal portion of the right paraglottic space (PGS). Tumor, which is seen with increased density, also extends towards the pre-epiglottic space (PES). Our CT observers concluded that the CT scans do not show obvious invasion of the epiglottic cartilage. T1 weighted MR scan (Fig. 2b) at the corresponding level shows tissue suspect for cancer, extending into the PES. Because of the close relation of tumor to the epiglottic cartilage, both MR observers concluded that there might be invasion of epiglottic cartilage. Microscopy confirmed that the epiglottic cartilage was invaded by cancer (not shown).

In six patients there were false negative CT interpretations and in another patient one false negative finding (Table 1). Of the six false negative CT examinations, five patients had (trans)glottic tumors (patients 4, 5, 6, 9, 12). Extension of the transglottic whether tumor into PES was underestimated, because the region around the epiglottic cartilage was seen with increased density nor was it enlarged by tumor. In contrast, MRI showed an abnormal intermediate signal intensity around the epiglottic cartilage.

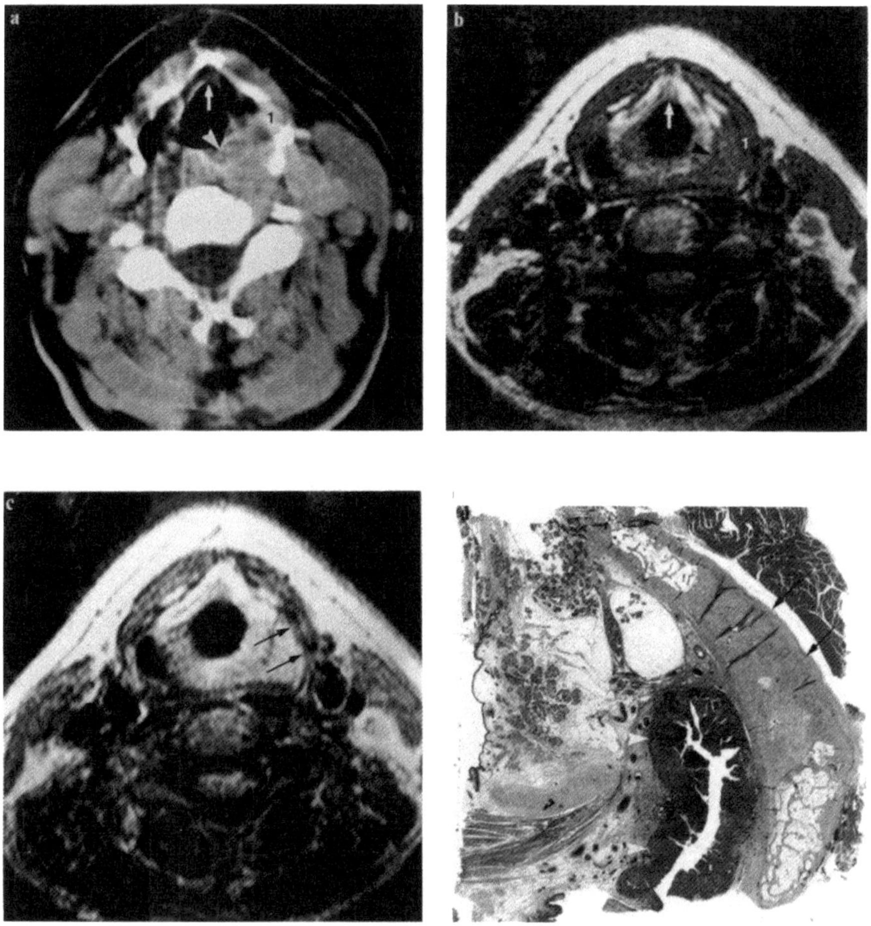

Figure 1. Case 16. Patient with a T2 hypopharyngeal lesion.
Figure 1a. Axial CT scan at a supraglottic level. Left piriform sinus is filled with tumor (arrowhead), which does not reach the area of the epiglottic cartilage (arrow).
Left thyroid lamina (1) may have been invaded by tumor or consist of non-ossified cartilage.
Figure 1b. Axial, T1 weighted MR examination (SE 400/38 ms) at a corresponding level shows tumor (arrowhead) with homogeneously intermediate signal intensity. It does not approach the epiglottic cartilage area (arrow), but borders the left thyroid lamina (1).
Figure 1c. Proton density examination (SE 1500/38 ms) at a corresponding level. Tumor, which is seen with increased signal intensity, has not invaded non-ossified cartilage (arrows), which is still seen with intermediate signal intensity.
Figure 1d. Left posterior quadrant of an axial sliced specimen. Microscopy shows tumor (arrowheads) bordering non-ossified cartilage (arrows).

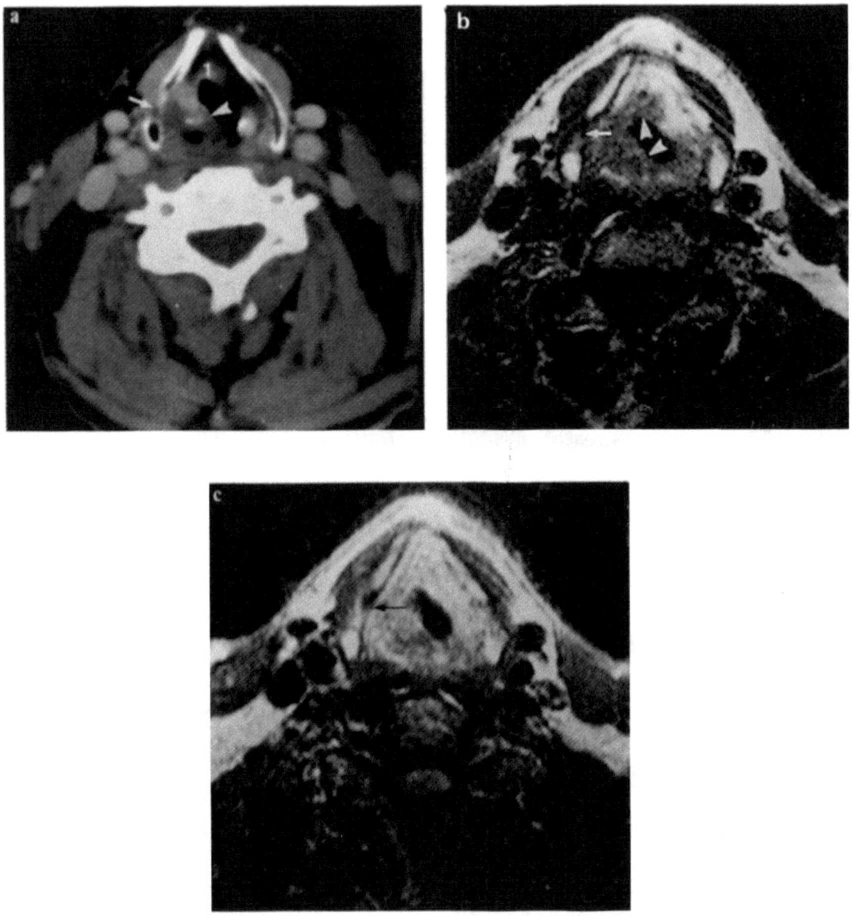

Figure 2. Case 4. Patient with a T3 transglottic lesion.
Figure 2a. Axial CT scan, just above level of the false cords.
Tumor (arrowhead) extends towards epiglottic cartilage (1), but no clear invasion is found. Thyroid cartilage is locally (arrow) seen with isodensity as tumor: tumor invasion or non-ossified cartilage.
Figure 2b. Axial, T1 weighted MR image (SE 400/38 ms) on a corresponding level shows tumor (arrowheads) invading the epiglottic cartilage. The medial wall of the thyroid cartilage is irregularly outlined (arrow).
Figure 2c. Proton density image (SE 1500/38 ms) demonstrates tumor with high contrast compared to non-ossified cartilage (arrow) which is still seen with intermediate signal intensity.

3.2. *Thyroid cartilage*

In Fig. 1a the thyroid cartilage is irregularly, but symmetrically calcified. Tumor abuts on the left thyroid lamina, which has partly an isodensity, suggestive of tumor invasion or of non-ossified cartilage. The CT observers concluded that invasion was absent. The T1 weighted MR examination (Fig. 1b) shows tumor, suspect for cancer, bordering the left thyroid lamina. The proton density image (Fig. 1c) shows tumorous tissue with increased signal intensity. The left thyroid lamina, adjacent to the tumor tissue, is still seen with intermediate signal intensity, indicating non-ossified cartilage. Malignant invasion is unlikely, due to its regularly outlined medial wall. Pathological examination (Fig. 1d) confirmed the MRI findings. In Fig. 2a, tumor approaches the right thyroid lamina, and irregularity of the right lamina is found. Cartilage invasion may not be proved definitely, because tumor tissue may border on non-ossified cartilage. Both CT observers concluded that there might be cartilage invasion. The corresponding T1 weighted MR examination (Fig. 2b) shows a suspect area in the right PGS. The tumor appears to border on non-ossified cartilage, because both the T1 weighted (Fig. 2b) and the proton density image (Fig. 2c) show thyroid cartilage, adjacent to tumor tissue, with intermediate signal intensity. The medial wall of the thyroid lamina is irregularly outlined. The MRI observers concluded that there might be invasion of non-ossified cartilage. Microscopy (not shown) demonstrated minor invasion of non-ossified cartilage.

An axial CT scan (Fig. 3a), at the level of the false cords in a male patient (No. 15) presenting with a T4 hypopharyngeal lesion, shows the right piriform sinus filled with a tumorous mass. The thyroid cartilage is almost entirely calcified. Because the medial wall of the right lamina shows a minimal irregularity adjacent to tumor tissue, one may conclude that minor invasion exists. Because, at a lower level, invasion of thyroid cartilage was more obvious, both CT observers agreed that invasion of the right lamina exists. On the corresponding T1 weighted MR scan (Fig. 3b), the pathological area

Figure 3. Case 15. Patient with T4 hypopharyngeal lesion.
Figure 3a. Axial CT scan at the level of the false cords.
Tumor borders right thyroid lamina (1). The medial wall of the lamina is irregularly outlined, suggesting minor cartilage invasion.
Figure 3b. Axial, T1 weighted examination (SE 400/38 ms) on a corresponding level shows right piriform sinus filled by a pathological mass. The dorsal extremity of the right thyroid lamina is seen with intermediate signal intensity (arrows).
Figure 3c. Axial, proton density image (SE 1500/38 ms) demonstrates that the dorsal extremity of the right thyroid lamina is invaded by tumor, the cortical rim being intact (arrow). Ventrally this area borders non-ossified cartilage (arrowhead) which is still seen with intermediate signal intensity.
Figure 3d. Microscopy of an axial sliced specimen confirms MR and contradicts CT findings. A large tumor mass infiltrates (arrows) the dorsal extremity of the right thyroid lamina. Ventrally to this area, non-ossified cartilage (arrowheads) is found which suggests cartilage invasion on the CT scan.

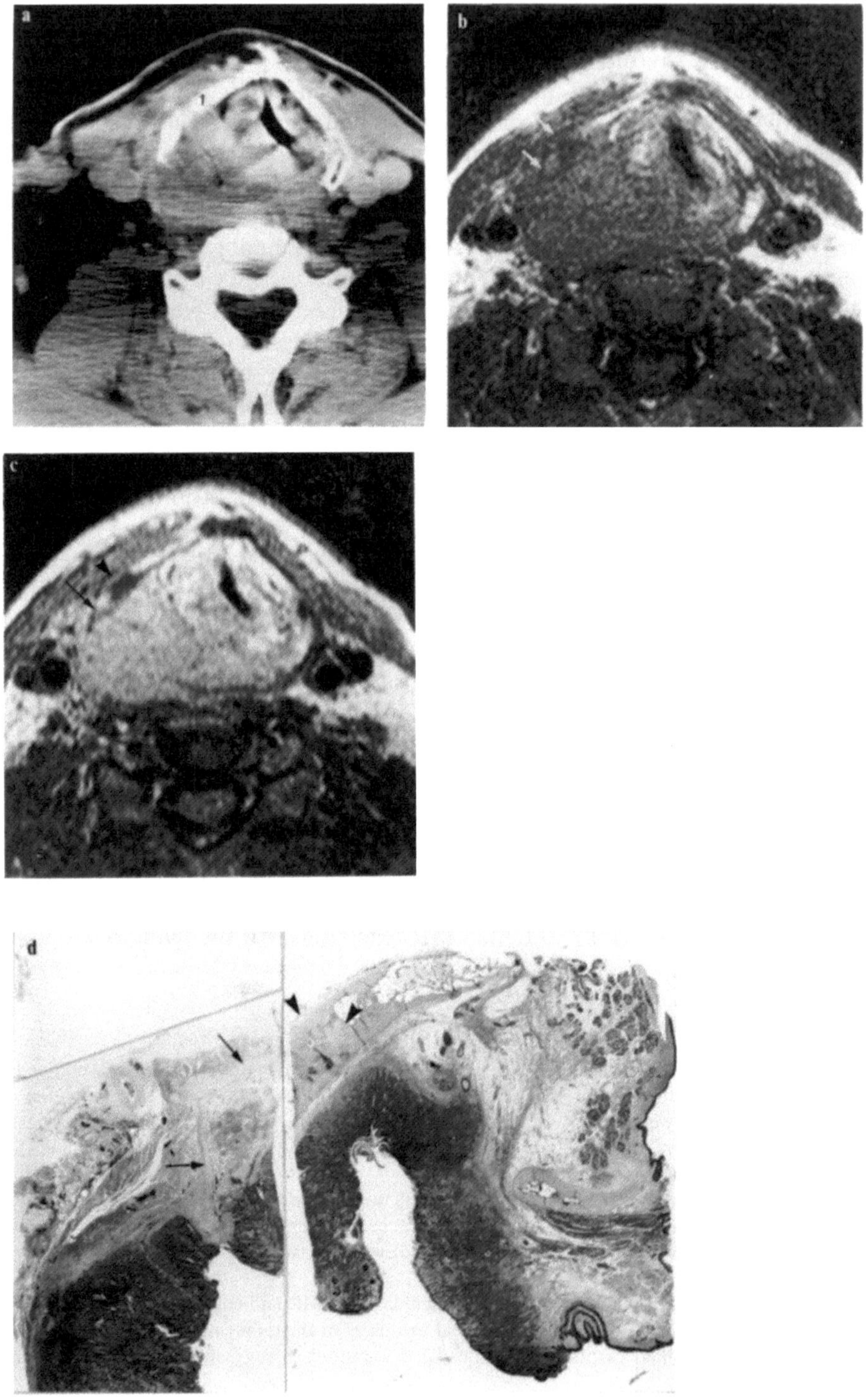

a
b
c
d

includes the dorsal portion of the right thyroid lamina. Fig. 3c (proton density image) shows that the entire pathological area has an increased signal intensity. Although the cortical rim is intact, the dorsal extreme of the right thyroid lamina appears to be invaded. Ventrally, this area borders on non-ossified cartilage, still being imaged with intermediate signal intensity. Microscopy (Fig. 3d) revealed that the dorsal extremity of the right thyroid lamina is invaded by pathological tissue: inflammatory and fibrous tissue with nests of cancer are present.

An axial CT scan (Fig. 4a), at the level of the false cords in a male patient (No. 5) with a glottic lesion, clinically staged as T3NO, demonstrates thickening of the dorsal portion of the left PGS, whereas the right compartment and the anterior commissure show no thickening. Thyroid cartilage is irregularly and asymmetrically calcified. Whereas tumor is found on the left side, the calcification pattern is more affected in the right thyroid lamina. Both CT observers concluded that invasion of the thyroid cartilage exists. On the T1 weighted MR image of the corresponding level (Fig. 4b), an intermediate signal area extends circumferentially around the laryngeal cavity, which is suggestive of cancer in both the right and left PGSs. Thyroid cartilage is found almost entirely with intermediate signal intensity, indicating non-ossified cartilage or cartilage invasion. The dorsal portion of the left thyroid lamina appears to be ossified and not invaded by tumor. On the proton density image (Fig. 4c), almost the whole area between the thin cortical layers of the right and left thyroid lamina has an increased signal

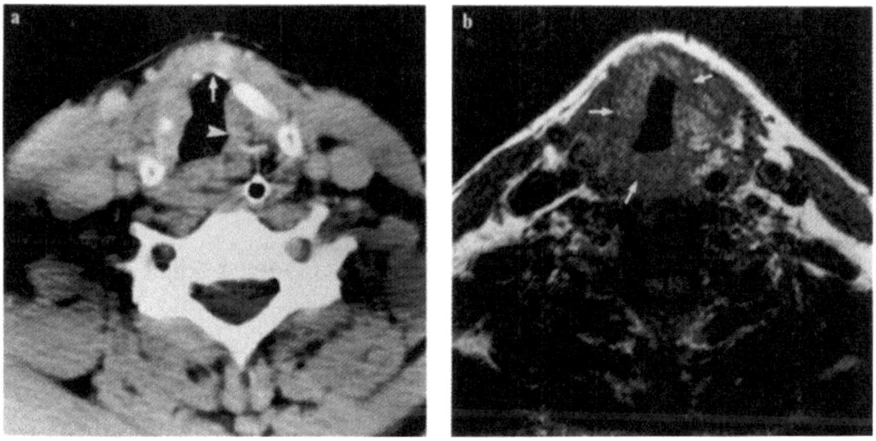

Figure 4. Case 5. Patient with T4 glottic lesion.

Figure 4a. Axial CT scan at the level of false cord. Tumor (arrowhead) is found in the dorsal portion of the left PGS. The right compartment and the anterior commissure (arrow) show no thickening. Whereas tumor is found on the left, calcification pattern is more affected in the right thyroid lamina.

Figure 4b. T1 weighted MR image (SE 400/38 ms) shows cancer (arrows) with homogeneously intermediate signal intensity, extending circumferentially around the walls of the laryngeal cavity.

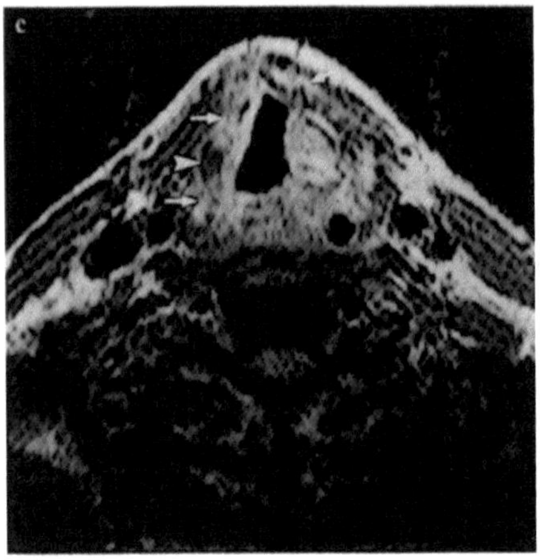

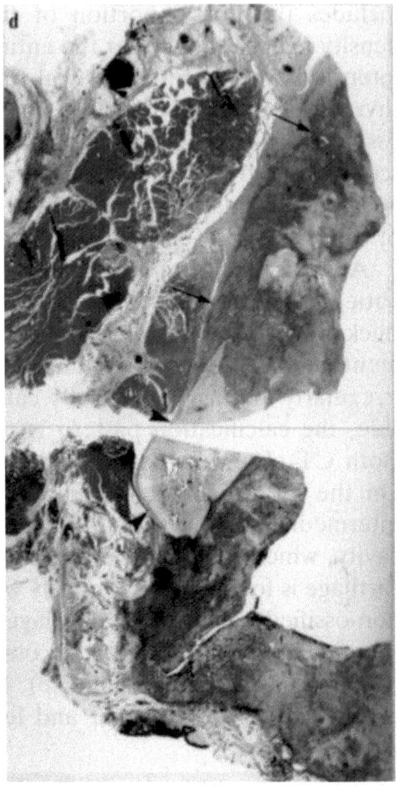

Figure 4c. The proton density image (SE 1500/38 ms) shows almost the entire area between the thin cortical layers (arrows) of both thyroid lamina with increased signal intensity, demonstrating cartilage invasion by pathological tissues. A small area of non-ossified cartilage (arrowhead) is still seen with intermediate signal intensity.
Figure 4d. Microscopic examination of the axial sliced right lamina confirms the greater part of the right lamina invaded by tumor (arrows). Non-ossified cartilage (arrowheads) is found in agreement with MRI findings.

intensity, representing invasion by pathological tissue. A small area in the right lamina still has intermediate signal intensity, indicating non-ossified cartilage. Microscopic examination of the right lamina (Fig. 4d) confirmed the MRI findings of invasion of the ventral and dorsal portions of the right lamina, being separated by normal and non-ossified cartilage.

There were four false negative diagnoses by CT and one false negative diagnosis by MRI (Table 1). All four false negative diagnosis by CT observers (Nos. 1, 3, 4, 12) were due to the intact contour of the calcified cartilages. In contrast, MRI showed invasion of bone marrow or showed an irregular outline of the medial wall of non-ossified thyroid cartilage. In one patient (No. 6), MRI failed to detect cartilage invasion due to movement artifacts on the proton density images. Both CT and MRI observers made one false positive interpretation in the same patient (No. 13).

3.3. *Arytenoid cartilage*

An axial CT scan (Fig. 5a) at the glottic level of the same patients as Fig. 4 shows thickening in the left PGS. No tumor was seen around the right arytenoid. It was stated by the CT observers that the left arytenoid is invaded by tumor and that the right arytenoid is intact. T1 weighted MR examination (Fig. 5b) demonstrates normal bone marrow of the left arytenoid, whereas the right arytenoid has an intermediate signal intensity. On the corresponding proton density examination (Fig. 5c), the area of the right arytenoid has an increased signal intensity, resulting from the invasion by pathological tissue. Microscopic examination of the left half confirmed the MRI findings that the left arytenoid was not invaded by cancer (Fig. 5d).

The failures of CT consisted of six false negative and two false positive diagnoses of invasion of the arytenoids. There were two false negative and three false positive interpretations of MRI examinations (Table 1). In five out of six CT false negative cases of invasion (Nos. 2, 6, 8, 9, 12), the arytenoid was neighbouring a tumor mass, but the calcification pattern and the contour of the cartilage was still intact. In contrast, MRI showed in this group, in all but one patient, a mass of intermediate signal intensity invading the marrow of the arytenoids. One false negative interpretation (No. 6) was made by the MRI observers, because in this case MRI did not show abnormality. In the patient (No. 5) of Fig. 5, a false positive and a false negative diagnosis by CT observers was caused by wrong interpretation of soft tissue swelling. Invasion of the right arytenoid of one patient (No. 14) was wrongly diagnosed by both CT and MRI observers. CT showed a hypodense arytenoid and MRI demonstrated an irregularly-shaped arytenoid among tumor tissue. In one patient (No. 8) the MRI observers made a false positive interpretation, because the arytenoid was found amid a large tumor mass. In a third false positive case (No. 13), microscopy showed fibrous tissue but no cancer in the arytenoid.

3.4. *Cricoid cartilage*

An axial CT scan at the subglottic level (Fig. 6a) of the same patient as shown in Fig. 3 (No. 15) demonstrated the right piriform sinus filled with a

Figure 5. Case 5. Patient with a T3 glottic lesion.
Figure 5a. Axial CT scan at the level of the glottis. The surroundings of the left arytenoid (arrowhead) are thickened, but no tumor is found in the area of the right arytenoid (arrow).
Figure 5b. Axial, T1 weighted scan (SE 400/38 ms) on a corresponding level shows that marrow of the left arytenoid (arrow) is not invaded by cancer, whereas the area around the right arytenoid has an intermediate signal intensity.
Figure 5c. Proton density scan (SE 1500/38 ms) demonstrates the area of the right arytenoid with increased signal intensity suggesting cartilage invasion.
Figure 5d. Microscopic examination of an axial sliced specimen confirms that the left arytenoid (1) is not invaded by cancer.

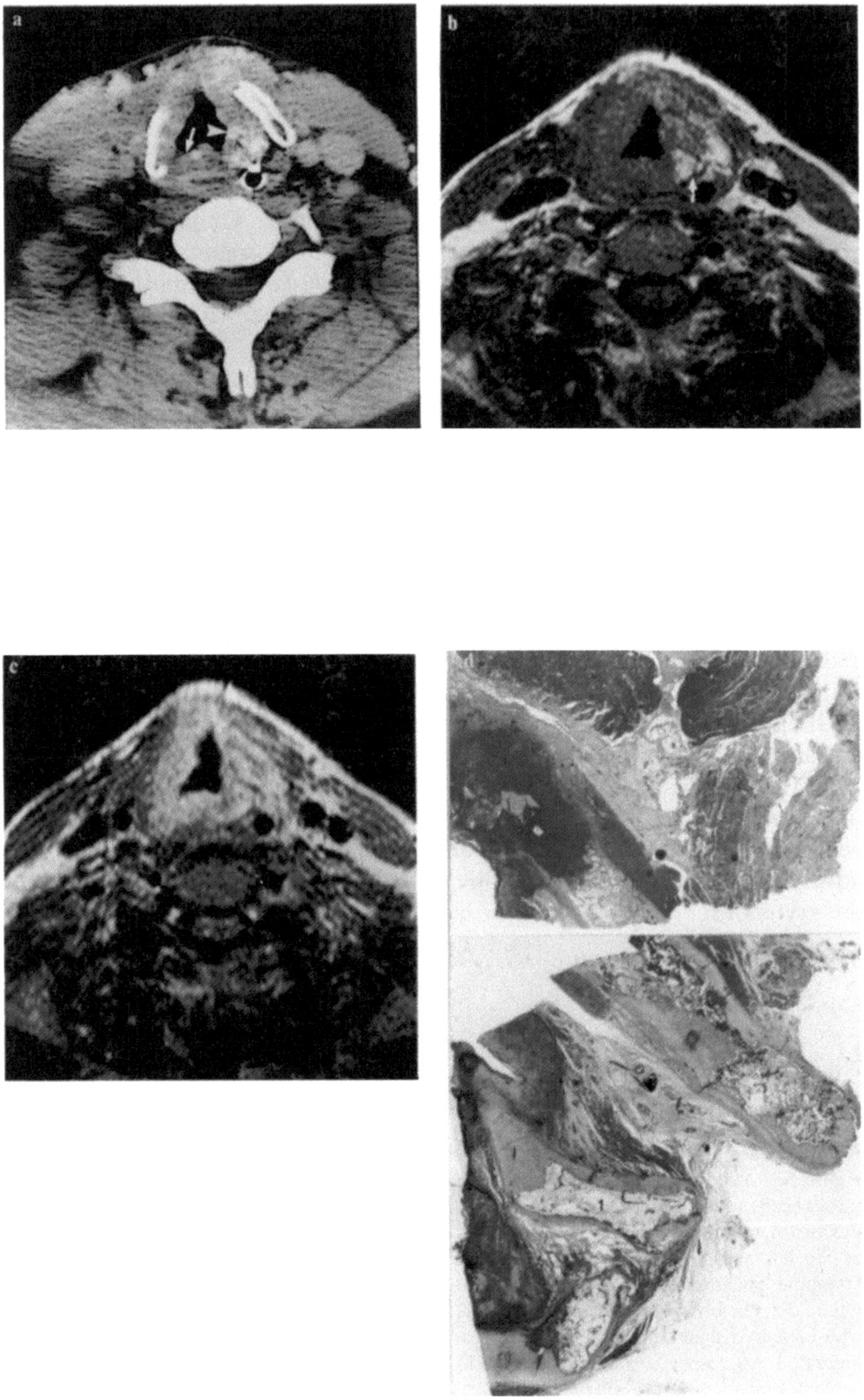
a
b
c
d

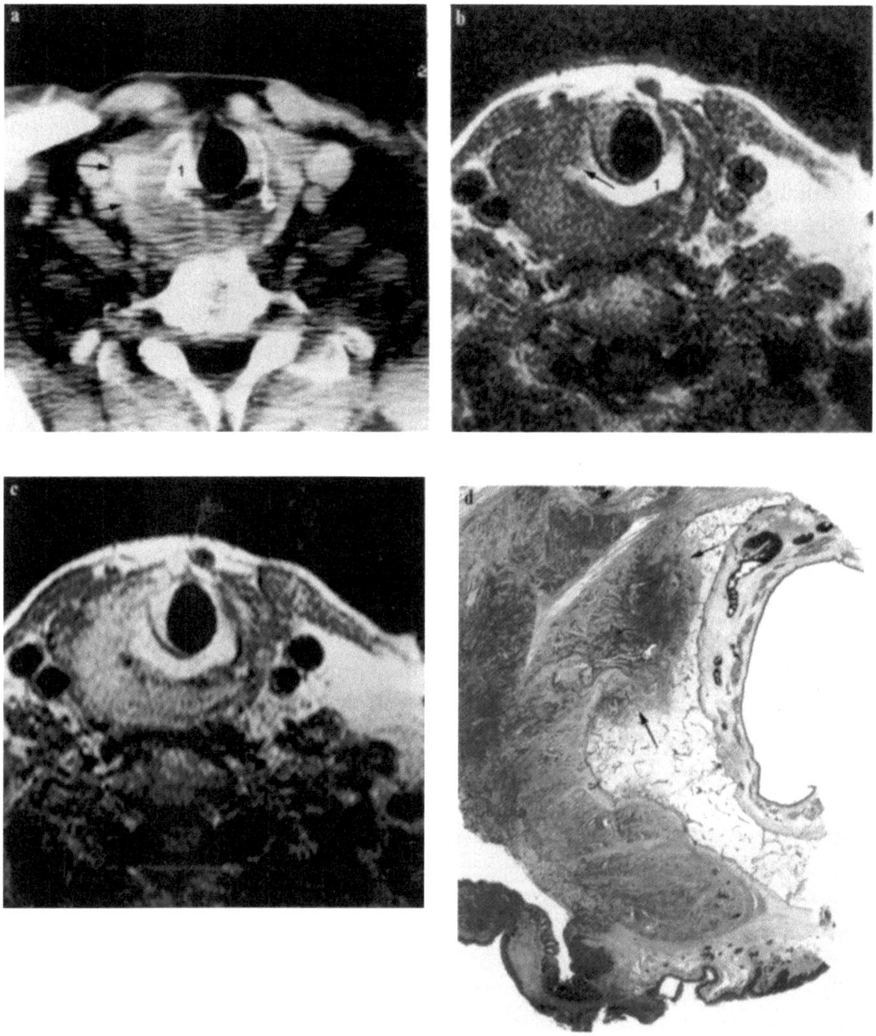

Figure 6. Case 15. Patient with a T4 hypopharyngeal lesion.

Figure 6a. Axial CT scan at the subglottic level. Large tumor (arrows) borders the cricoid (1), but no invasion is found.

Figure 6b. Axial, T1 weighted examination (SE 400/38 ms) at a corresponding level. Minor invasion (arrow) of the bone marrow of the cricoid (1) is found.

Figure 6c. Axial, proton density examination (SE 1500/38 ms) shows entire tumor mass with increased signal intensity.

Figure 6d. Microscopic study of the axial sliced right part of the cricoid confirms MR finding of invasion (arrow) of the cricoid (1).

large tumorous mass. The cricoid has a calcified rim, but no obvious invasion is found. MR images (Fig. 6b and c) demonstrated minor invasion into the right border of the cricoid. Microscopic study confirmed the MRI findings (Fig. 6d). Whereas CT examinations of 4 patients were false negatively diagnosed, MRI observers made no false negative interpretation. In 3 out of 4 patients (Nos. 8, 9, 15) CT did not show invasion of the cricoid, because the calcification pattern and the contour of the cricoid were intact, or showed locally even more calcification. In contrast, MRI showed invasion of the bone marrow of the ossified cricoid. In one patient (No. 5) the CT observers made a false positive interpretation, because the tumor was left-sided, whereas the calcification pattern was affected on the right side. Both CT and MRI observers made one false positive interpretation of the same patient (No. 7). An asymmetrical cricoid, bordering on a large tumor, caused a false positive interpretation on both CT and MR images.

3.5. *Group of patients for which no pathologic correlation was available*

Figure 7a shows an axial CT scan at the glottic level of a patient with a T2NO glottic lesion. Both arytenoids appeared not to be invaded, because the contour of both arytenoids was intact. In contrast, MR examinations (Figs. 7b and c) demonstrated obvious invasion of the right arytenoid. On an axial CT scan at the high subglottic level of the same patient (Fig. 8a), a tumor was found, adjacent to the anterior commissure, but the thyroid cartilage appeared to be normal and calcified. The T1 weighted MR examin-

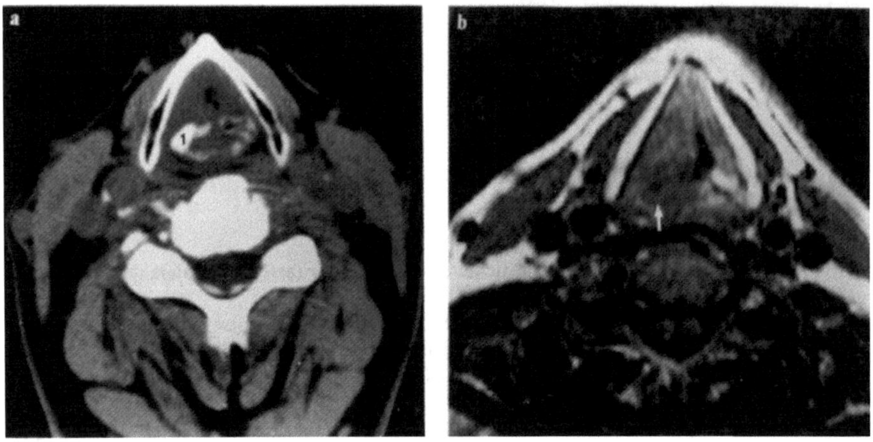

Figure 7. Patient with T2 glottic lesion.
Figure 7a. Axial CT scan at the glottic level. No obvious invasion of the right arytenoid (1) exists.
Figure 7b. Axial, T1 weighted examination (SE 400/38 ms) shows right arytenoid with intermediate signal intensity (arrow).

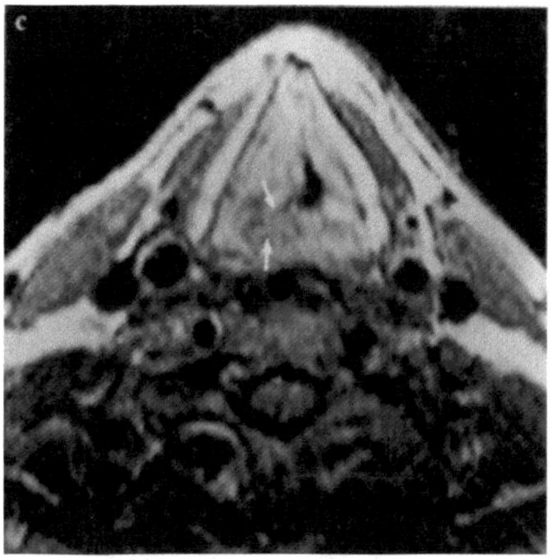

Figure 7c. Axial, proton density examination (SE 1500/38 ms) shows bone marrow (arrows) in the right arytenoid with increased signal intensity which strenghtens the suspicion of cartilage invasion.

ation (Fig. 8b) suggested invasion of the anterior commissure and the right portion of the cricoid. Proton density and T2 weighted images (Fig. 8d even more than Fig. 8c) demonstrated that both regions were invaded by tumor.

In this group of patients the CT readers observed evident cartilage invasion in 2 out of 26 patients, whereas the MRI observers concluded that in 6 patients one or more cartilages were evidently invaded.

3.6. *Movement Artifacts*

Whereas the CT observers concluded that adequate interpretation of all scans was possible, the MRI observers thought that the presence of movement artifacts interfered with adequate diagnosis in 7 out of 42 examinations. Four out of seven patients had chronic respiratory disease, or severe dyspnea in their histories. Only four patients in the remaining group of 35 had chronic respiratory disease.

4. Discussion

The laryngeal skeleton consists of two types of cartilages. The epiglottic cartilage consists of elastic cartilage and in general does not ossify. The cricoid, the thyroid cartilage, and the greater part of the arytenoids consist of hyaline cartilage and ossify. Often, the process of ossification and calcification is very irregular. Detection of cartilage invasion is of great clinical importance. Complications due to irradiation treatment frequently occur in

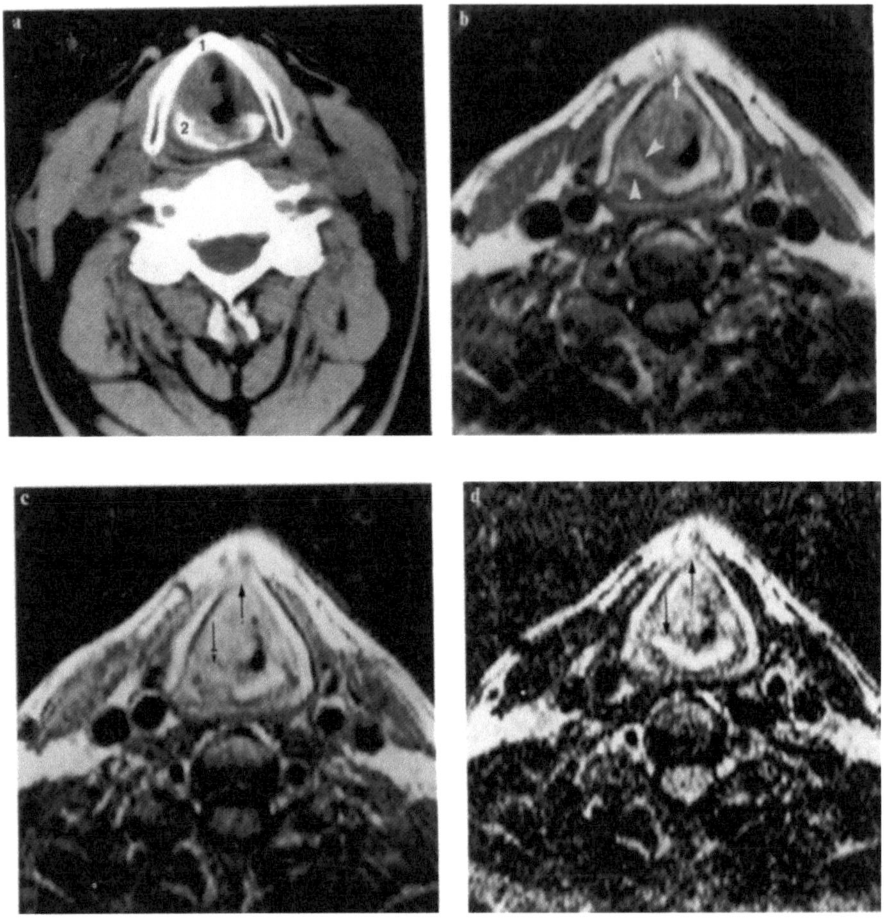

Figure 8. Patient with a T2 glottic lesion.

Figure 8a. An axial CT scan at a high subglottic level. Tumor is found narrowing the intralaryngeal lumen. Both thyroid (1) and cricoid (2) cartilages do not show obvious cartilage invasion.

Figure 8b. T1 weighted MR image (SE 400/38 ms) suggests invasion of the right half of the cricoid cartilage (arrowheads) and the anterior commissure (arrows).

Figure 8c. Proton density image (SE 1500/38 ms). The bone marrow of both thyroid and cricoid cartilages (arrows) is seen with increased signal intensity.

Figure 8d. T2 weighted images (SE 1500/76 ms) demonstrate tumor, invading the cartilages (arrows), with even more signal intensity, indicating invasion by tumor.

the presence of cartilage invasion. Demonstration of such an invasion may contribute to better selection between irradiation treatment and surgery [1].

Partial laryngectomy is contraindicated if the cartilages have undergone invasion by tumor [12].

4.1. *Elastic cartilage: epiglottic cartilage*

In the present study, invasion of the epiglottic cartilage was frequently false positively diagnosed, due to underestimation of the extension of tumor tissue into the PES. In contrast with earlier expectations [13,14], MRI observers succeeded very well in detecting invasion of the epiglottic cartilage. T1 weighted images show tumor in high contrast with surrounding fat, normally present at the supraglottic level (Figs. 1b, 2b). Although the epiglottic cartilage is not always recognizable, the vicinity of tumor to the area of the epiglottic cartilage appears to be very suspicious for cartilage invasion. In contrast, if surrounding tissues of the epiglottic cartilage are seen with normally high signal intensity, invasion of the cartilage can be excluded (Fig. 1b). Proton density images have little value for detection of invasion of the epiglottic cartilage, because contrast between pathological tissue and fat is minimal (Fig. 1c, 2c).

4.2. *Hyaline cartilage: thyroid, cricoid and arytenoid cartilages*

The changes in hyaline cartilages have been the subject of much discussion. Roncallo has reviewed the literature on this subject [15]. Some authors consider ossification and calcification to be the same processes, whereas others maintain that calcification precedes ossification. Roncallo himself favours the view, originally put forward by Chievitz, that the two processes are absolutely independent of each other [15, 16].

The CT appearance of normal hyaline cartilages is mainly determined by the state of calcification. The hyaline cartilages may be variably composed of calcified and non-calcified cartilage, or of bone with a marrow cavity [17]. Uncalcified cartilage and bone marrow are much less well displayed on CT than calcified cartilage. The cortical rim of ossified cartilage with relatively abundant marrow may appear thinner than ossified cartilage, containing extensive bony trabeculae within the marrow cavity. Its margin may be indistinct [18].

The MR image of hyaline cartilages correlates very well with the histological appearance: the process of endochondral ossification. As previously described, both T1 weighted and proton density images show non-ossified cartilage with intermediate signal intensity [9]. Both types of images show ossified cartilage with a typically three-layer appearance: bone marrow showing high signal intensity and the bony rims having low signal intensity [5,9,14].

Cancer preferably invades ossified cartilage. Very frequently CT fails severely in detecting invasion of calcified thyroid, cricoid and arytenoid cartilages (Figs. 3a, 6a, 7a, 8a, etc.). The contour or pattern of calcification does not show deformities, whereas in some cases invaded cartilage is even seen with increased density. In all ossified cartilages, tumor may grossly invade the medullary space of the laryngeal cartilages, and may not be detected by CT if the surrounding bone is still intact. Tumor growth infiltrating the marrow cavity without destroying bony trabeculae or surrounding bone may escape detection because the presence of these bony structures enables reconstruction of an apparently normal cartilage on CT. In contrast, MRI is capable of showing early invasion of ossified cartilage. On T1 weighted images invasion of bone marrow is found with intermediate signal intensity (Figs. 3b, 6b, 7b, 8b).

In some patients CT may suggest invasion of cartilage (Figs. 2a, 3a). Because uncalcified or poorly calcified cartilage may not be well displayed by CT, so erosion or destruction may be simulated. By contrast, proton density MR images are capable of differentiating between invaded bone marrow and non-ossified cartilage (Figs. 2c, 3c), by showing tumor with increased signal intensity. Sometimes, CT fails in detecting invasion of the arytenoid and cricoid, because no tumor was found around these cartilages (Figs. 4a, 5a). On CT, usual indicators of tumor are thickening of soft tissue structures, distortion or displacement of the adjacent lumen, and the presence of an area with mostly increased density [18]. Cancer localisation is not always possible by CT, and sometimes detracts from an assessment of the real extent of tumor spread. MRI has greater possibilities than CT for the assessment of the site and the extension of tumor [14] (Figs. 4b, 5b).

In a minority of cases cancer invades non-ossified cartilage. Whereas cancer spreads rapidly in bone marrow of ossified cartilage after invading through the cortical rim, infiltration of non-ossified cartilage occurs gradually. Contrast between non-ossified cartilage and tumor is higher on proton density images than it is on T1 weighted images. The probability of invasion of non-ossified cartilage increases, if an irregularity of non-ossified cartilage adjacent to tumor is found on proton density images (Fig. 2c).

Because diagnosis of cartilage invasion may result in laryngectomy, evaluation of false positive interpretations of MR images is most important. The MRI observers made five false positive diagnoses of cartilage invasion. In one patient (No. 13), the MRI readers observed invasion in an arytenoid, which was filled with fibrous tissue. The four other false positive diagnoses were due to different reasons: difficult interpretation of invasion of non-ossified cartilage, low signal-to-noise ratio of some proton density images, irregularities of cartilages and movement artifacts.

The previous discussion indicates that "probable" and "evident" cartilage invasion, as shown by MRI, are good parameters for the detection of cartilage invasion and that "no" and "probably no" cartilage invasion, as shown by MRI, are good parameters for the absence of cartilage invasion. MRI findings in those patients treated by surgery would raise the clinical stage of all but three patients. To calculate the accuracy of the detection of cartilage invasion, the numbers of "probable" and "evident" cartilage invasions were summarized, and so were the numbers of "probably no" and "no" cartilage invasion. In our experience, specificities (percentage of cases in which the absence of cartilage invasion was correctly diagnosed) of CT and MRI for detecting invasion of the laryngeal cartilages are approximately equal, 39/43 = 91% and 38/43 = 88%, respectively. CT has a much lower sensitivity (percentage of cases in which the presence of cartilage invasion was correctly diagnised) than MRI, 17/37 = 46% and 33/37 = 89%, respectively.

We recommend MRI as the modality of choice for the diagnosis of cartilage invasion. If diagnostic use of MRI examinations of, for instance, patients with chronic respiratory disease is impossible as a result of movement artifacts (in our hands 16% of the cases), then CT will be necessary.

5. Summary

MRI is superior to CT in detecting invasion of the laryngeal cartilages. Frequently calcified cartilage, invaded by cancer, is found on CT with an intact contour and intact calcification pattern. Tumor tissue bordering on non-calcified cartilage may simulate cartilage invasion. In contrast, MRI offers clear criteria for the demonstration or exclusion of cartilage invasion. This results in a specificity equal to CT, and a much higher sensitivity. The existence of movement artifacts interfered with adequate diagnosis in 16% of the MRI examinations.

References

1. Gerritsen GJ, Valk J, van Velzen DJ, Snow GB. Computed tomography: a mandatory investigational procedure for the T-staging of advanced laryngeal cancer. Clin Otolaryngol 1986;11:307–316.
2. Yeager VL, Lawson C, Archer CR. Ossification of laryngeal cartilages as it relates to computed tomography. Invest Radiol 1982;17:11–19.
3. Hoover LA, Calcaterra TC, Walter GA, Larsson SG. Preoperative CT scan evaluation for laryngeal carcinoma: correlation with pathological findings. Laryngoscope 1984;94:310–315.
4. Decker JW, Price JC, Goldstein JC. Advanced laryngeal cancer. Relevance of pathologic stage to survival and therapy. Arch Otolaryngol Head Neck Surg 1986;112:1163–1167.
5. McArdle CB, Bailey BJ, Amparo EG. Surface coil magnetic resonance imaging of the normal larynx. Arch Otolaryngol Head Neck Surg 1986;112:616–622.
6. Castelijns JA, Doornbos J, Verbeeten B Jr., Vielvoye GJ, Bloem JL. Magnetic resonance imaging of the normal larynx. J Comput Assist Tomogr 1985;9(5):919–25.
7. Lufkin RB, Hanafee WN. Application of surface coils to MR anatomy of the larynx. AJNR 1985;6:491–497.
8. Lufkin RB, Hanafee WN, Wortham D, Hoover L. Larynx and hypopharynx: MR imaging with surface coils. Radiology 1986;158:747–754.

9. Castelijns JA, Gerritsen GJ, Kaiser MC, Valk J, Jansen W, Meyer CJLM, Snow GB. MRI of laryngeal cartilages, normal or invaded by primary cancer; MRI-histopathologic correlation. Laryngoscope 1987;97:1085–1093.
10. Castelijns JA. Laryngeal cancer. In: Valk J, ed. Magnetic Resonance Imaging of the brain, head, neck and spine- a teaching atlas of clinical applications. Dordrecht: Martinus Nijhoff Publishers, 1987.
11. Michaels L, Gregor RT. Examination of the larynx in the histopathology laboratory. J Clin Pathol 1980; 33:705–709.
12. Moss WT, Brand WN, Battifora H. The endolarynx, hypopharynx, and thyroid. In: Moss WT, ed. Radiation Oncology. Saint Louis: The C.V. Mosby Compagny, 1973;195–232.
13. Castelijns JA, Valk J, Kaiser MC, Gerritsen GJ, Jansen W, Snow GB. MRI of laryngeal tumors. In: RSNA Scientific Program of the 72nd Scientific Assembly and Annual Meeting. 1986:366.
14. Castelijns JA, Kaiser MC, Valk J, Gerritsen GJ, van Hattum AH, Snow GB. MRI of laryngeal cancer. J Comput Assist Tomogr 1987;11(1):134–140.
15. Roncallo, P. Researches about ossification and confirmation of the thyroid cartilage in men. Acta Otolaryng 1948;36:110–134.
16. Chievitz JH. Untersuchungen ueber die verknocherung der menschlichen kehllnorpel. Arch anat uentwickelingsgesch 1882;4:200–208.
17. Sagel SS, Aufderheide JF, Aronberg DJ, Stanley RJ, Archer CR. High resolution computed tomography in the staging of carcinoma of the larynx. The Laryngoscope 1981;91,292–300.
18. Archer CR, Yeager VL. Computed tomography of laryngeal cancer with histopathological correlation. Laryngoscope 1982;92:1173–1180.

Chapter 10: MR findings of cartilage invasion by laryngeal cancer. Value in predicting outcome of radiation therapy

Authors: J.A. Castelijns, M.D. (1)
R.P. Golding, F.R.C.R. (1)
C. van Schaik, M.D. (1)
J. Valk, M.D. (1)
G.B. Snow, M.D. (2)

(1) Dept. of Radiology
(2) Dept. of Otolaryngology

Institution: Free University Hospital
Amsterdam
The Netherlands

Abstract

Thirty nine patients who had underwent radiotherapy with a curative intent for laryngeal cancer were examined before treatment by magnetic resonance (MR) imaging, between November 1985 and to January 1987. MR findings of cartilage invasion were correlated with the effectiveness of radiation treatment. Adequate interpretation of the MR examinations was not possible in four cases (10%). Cartilage invasion was found in 16 out of the 35 remaining patients and was found even in small glottic lesions, clinically staged as T1b and T2. Laryngeal cancer recurred in 10 of the 16 patients with cartilage invasion shown by MR imaging. The presence of even small foci of invasion of the thyroid cartilage by laryngeal cancer appeared to increase the subsequent risk of tumor recurrence. Cartilage invasion seen at MR imaging might therefore shift the preference to partial laryngectomy as the initial treatment for small glottic tumors. Alternatively, radiation therapy alone would appear to require stringent follow-up to detect possible recurrence.

1. Introduction

Invasion of the laryngeal cartilages by cancer has a bearing on the effectiveness of radiation therapy [1–4]. Complications, such as severe edema and radionecrosis, mainly occur in cases of highly fractionated treatment or high total dose when invasion of bone or cartilage is present [2, 4–6]. Recently, however, the inability of radiation therapy to cure laryngeal cancer involving bone or cartilage has been questioned by Million [7].

Computer tomography (CT) has the capacity to demonstrate submucosal tumor spread and gross cartilage invasion, but it fails to detect early cartilage invasion [8]. Nevertheless, a recent report stated that CT evidence of cartilage invasion can be useful as a predictor of an unfavorable response to radiation therapy [9].

Magnetic resonance (MR) imaging displays laryngeal anatomy in great detail, especially non-ossified and ossified cartilage [10]. Recent work, in which MR images were compared with pathological specimens, has shown that MRI has the ability to demonstrate even minor cartilage invasion [11]. Although MRI is more sensitive than CT in detecting cartilage invasion, there is clearly a lower limit of detectable cartilage invasion on MR imaging. Criteria for detection of cartilage invasion have been developed [11, 12].

With the combined use of T1 weighted and proton density transverse images, MR imaging is of great value in the diagnostic work-up of cartilage invasion in previously untreated patients.

The aim of this study was to correlate MR findings regarding cartilage invasion, applying the criteria mentioned above, with the effectiveness of radiation treatment. In addition, the risk of recurrence was investigated in relation to the clinical staging of the tumor and the site and extent of cartilage invasion.

2. Materials and methods

Thirty-nine patients, seen from November 1985 through January 1987, having previously untreated laryngeal carcinomas, were investigated by MR imaging prior to radiation therapy administered with the intent to cure. Treatment was performed with megavoltage radiation by left-to-right fields. the size of the treatment field depended on the T-stage, extent of the primary tumor and the presence of the probability of lymphatic spread. The extent of the tumor volume, the degree of differentiation and the rate of regression of the tumor during radiation treatment each influenced the total dose (6250 to 7600 cGy). The MR findings did not influence the radiation doses.

Adequate interpretation was possible in 35 patients. Their ages ranged from 43 to 88 years. There were 31 men and 4 women. All patients had squamous cell carcinoma. Further data are presented in Table 1. All MR examinations were obtained within 4 weeks before the beginning of the radiation treatment. The mean follow-up after the end of radiation treatment was 24 months. To avoid bias caused by patient selection, our MR series was a consecutive one, although patients who had received a cardiac pacemaker or who were in a poor clinical condition were excluded.

MR images were obtained with a 0.6 Tesla superconductive system (Teslacon I; Technicare, Cleveland, Ohio) with a half saddle-shaped surface coil placed around the anterior aspect of the neck as a receiver antenna. A multisection two-dimensional Fourier transform spin-echo (SE) pulse sequence was used in all cases. In sagittal, transverse, and frontal planes, a T1 weighted technique was used, with a repetition time (TR) of 200–400 ms and an echo time (TE) of 38 ms. In the axial plane, we also generated proton-density images (SE 1500/38[TR ms/TE ms]) and T2 weighted images (SE 1500/76) at each corresponding level. The acquisition of T1 weighted images was repeated four times for signal averaging, and the acquisition of proton-density and T2 weighted images was repeated twice. A 4 mm section thickness was used, with a 3 mm intersection gap. The field of view was kept as small as possible (200 × 200 mm), so that with a 256 × 192 acquisition matrix, T1 weighted images had a pixel resolution of 0.8 × 1.0 mm. Proton-density images and T2 weighted images had a 256 × 128 acquisition matrix. Acqui-

Table 1. Patient data: location and stage of tumor, invasion of cartilage, and tumor recurrence

Patient No.	Location*	Stage		Invasion†					Local Recurrence
		T	N	TC	CC	LA	RA	Site	
1	Sup	2	0	–	–	–	–	...	0
2	Sup	4	0	+n	–	–	+n	1, 3	1
3	Glottic	2	1	+o	–	–	–	1	1
4	Glottic	1b	0	+o	–	–	–	1	1‡
5	Glottic	1a	0	–	–	–	–	...	0
6	Glottic	1a	0	–	–	–	–	...	0
7	Glottic	1a	0	–	–	–	–	...	0
8	Glottic	4	0	+o	+o	+o	–	1, 3	1
9	Glottic	1b	0	+o	–	–	–	1	1
10	Sup	3	1	+o	–	–	–	4	1‡
11	Glottic	1a	0	–	–	–	–	...	0
12	Glottic	1a	0	–	–	–	–	...	0
13	Glottic	2	0	–	–	–	–	...	1
14	Glottic	2	2	+o	–	–	–	1	0
15	Glottic	2	0	–	–	–	–	...	0
16	Glottic	2	0	–	–	–	–	...	0
17	Glottic	1a	0	+o	–	–	–	1	0
18	Sub	4	0	+o	+o	+o	–	1, 3	0
19	Glottic	3	0	–	+n	–	+n	3	0
20	Glottic	2	0	+o	–	–	–	1	1
21	Glottic	1a	0	–	–	–	–	...	0
22	Glottic	1a	0	–	–	–	–	...	0
23	Glottic	1b	0	+o	–	–	–	1	0
24	Sup	1	0	–	–	–	–	...	0
25	Sup	3	0	–	–	–	–	...	0
26	Glottic	2	0	–	–	–	–	...	0
27	Glottic	1b	0	–	–	–	–	...	0
28	Sup	4	0	–	–	–	–	...	0
29	Glottic	2	0	+o	–	–	–	1	1
30	Glottic	2	2	+n	–	–	–	1, 2	0
31	Glottic	2	0	–	–	–	–	...	0
32	Glottic	2	0	+o	+o	–	+o	1, 3	1
33	Glottic	2	0	–	–	–	–	...	1
34	Glottic	4	0	+o	+o	+o	–	1, 3	1
35	Glottic	3	0	–	–	–	–	...	0

* Location of primary tumor. Sup = supraglottic, Sub = subglottic.

† TC = thyroid cartilage, CC = cricoid cartilage, LA = left arytenoid, RA = right arytenoid, minus sign = no cartilage invasion, +n = invasion of nonossified cartilage, +o = invasion of ossified cartilage. Site 1 = area under anterior commissure, 2 = lower edge of the thyroid lamina, 3 = cricoarytenoid joint, 4 = thyroid cartilage elsewhere.

‡ Regional recurrence also occurred in patients 4 and 10.

sition times varied from 3 to 6 minutes. Patients were instructed to breathe quietly and to refrain from swallowing.

All pretreatment MR studies were reviewed by two independent observers (R.P.G., C.v.S) in order to assess invasion of the thyroid, cricoid and arytenoid cartilage. The reviewers were trained in evaluating MR examinations. T1 weighted images allow separation between pathological bone marrow, which is found with intermediate signal intensity, and normal bone marrow, which is seen with high signal intensity. Proton-density images permit differentiation between nonossified cartilage, which is seen with intermediate signal intensity, and tumor tissue, which is found with increased signal intensity compared to T1 weighted images. Invasion of non-ossified cartilage was concluded to be present if the margin of non-ossified cartilage showed irregularity. The observers were blind to previous interpretations of the studies, clinical information, and therapeutic decisions. At the end of the first set of readings, the reviewers compared their findings. In cases of discord, both reviewers of each modality considered the examinations together in order to reach a consensus where possible. The radiological findings are presented in Table 1. The reviewers were asked if adequate interpretation of the images was possible. This was chiefly to take account of movement artifacts, but other causes of image degradation were also noted.

3. Results

There were six cases of disagreement between the observers, in which one reviewer interpreted the study as indicating probable or evident cartilage invasion and the other one believed there was probably no or definitely no invasion.

Data regarding the presence of cartilage invasion and the subsequent occurrence of recurrent cancer are presented in Table 1. Both observers concluded that adequate interpretation was not possible in four of 39 patients (approximately 10%). These examinations were excluded from further study. MR imaging demonstrated cartilage invasion in 16 out of 35 patients (13 men and 3 women). Thyroid cartilage was involved in 15 patients. In the thyroid cartilage of 11 patients most of whom had T1b and T2 glottic lesions, only a small part of the thyroid cartilage in the area of the anterior commissure was involved (Figs. 1–3). In one patient the inferior edge of the thyroid lamina was involved (patient 30). In five patients, the cricoid cartilage was invaded. In one of these five (patient 19), only the cricoid and arytenoid cartilages were suspected, and no invasion of the thyroid cartilage was found. In six patients, invasion of at least one arytenoid cartilage was suspected. In patients with suspected invasion of the arytenoid and/or cricoid cartilage, infiltration of cartilage around the crico-arytenoid joint was found (Figs. 2, 3). At least two cartilages were involved in six patients. Ossified cartilage

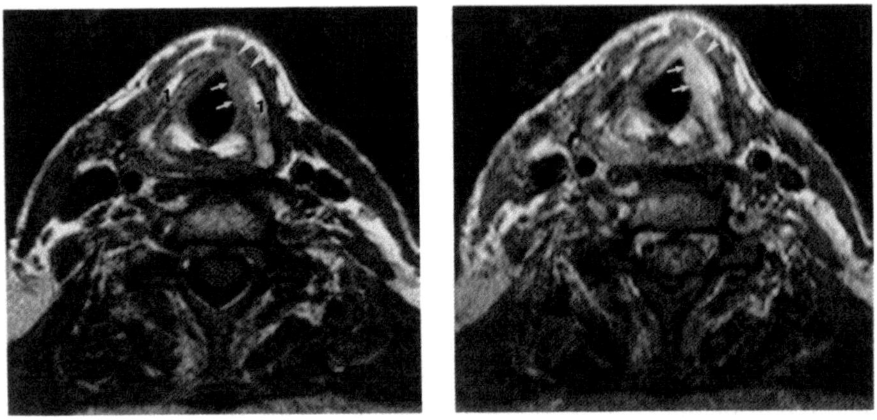

Figure 1. Patient 23. MR images of a patient with a stage T1b glottic lesion. (a) Axial T1 weighted image (SE 400/38) at the true cord level shows tumor (arrows) in the anterior two-thirds of the left vocal cord, the anterior commissure and the anterior part of the right vocal cord. Invasion (arrowheads) of the thyroid cartilage (1) in the area of the anterior commissure is seen. (b) Axial proton-density image (SE 1500/38) demonstrates tumor tissue (arrows) with slightly increased signal intensity compared with the T1 weighted image, confirming cartilage invasion (arrowheads).

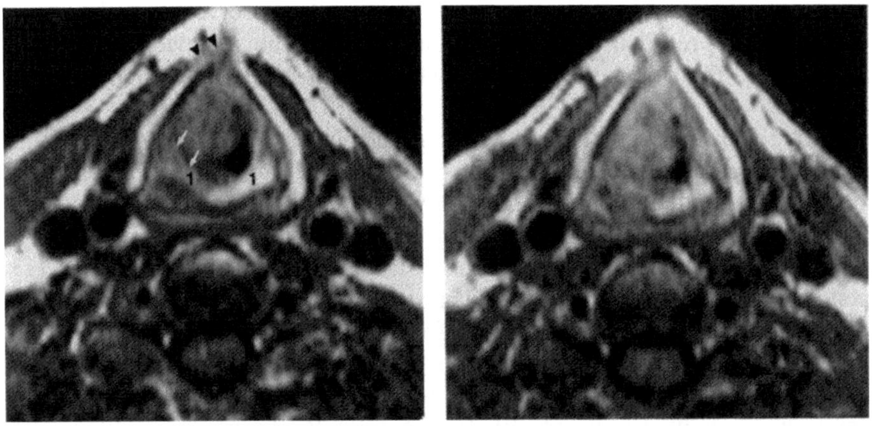

Figure 2. Patient 32. MR images of a patient with a stage T2 glottic lesion. (a) On the axial T1 weighted image (SE 400/38) at the glottic level, tumor is seen narrowing the intralaryngeal lumen. Tumor invasion (arrows) of the right half of the cricoid cartilage (1) and in the anterior commissure (arrowheads) of the thyroid cartilage is suggested. (b) On the proton density image (SE 1500/38) at the corresponding level, the invaded marrow of both cricoid and thyroid cartilages has slightly increased signal intensity compared with the T1 weighted image, confirming cartilage invasion.

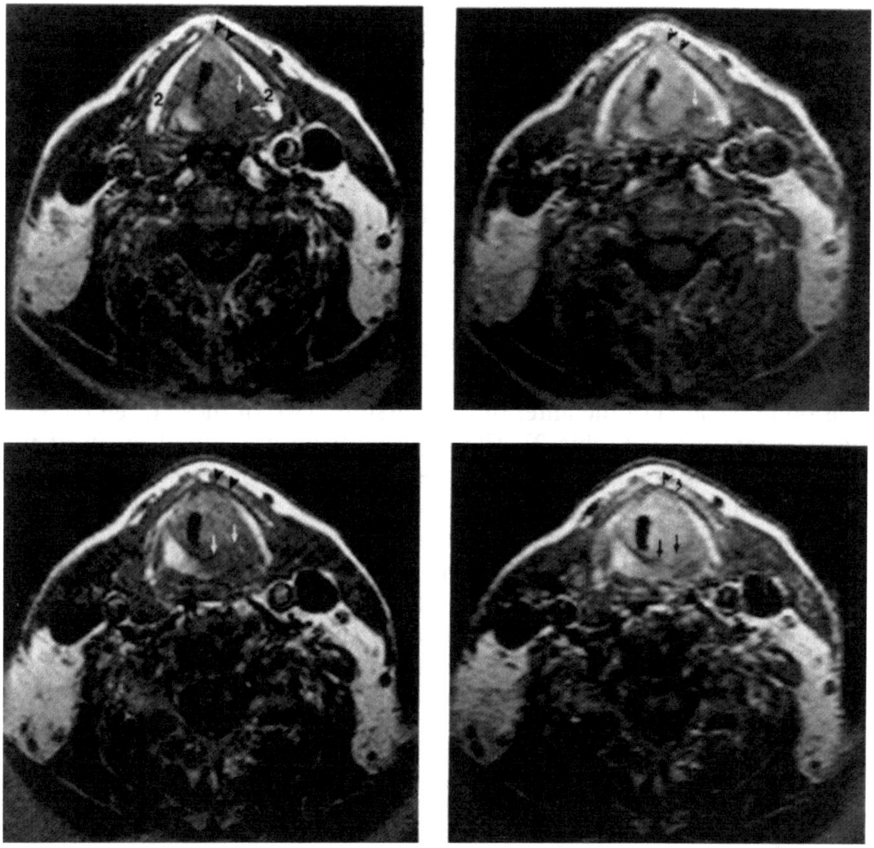

Figure 3. Patient 34. MR images in a patient with a T4 glottic lesion. (a) Axial T1 weighted image (SE 400/38) at false cord level shows invasion (arrows) of the left arytenoid (1) and in the anterior commissure (arrowheads) of the thyroid cartilage (2). (b) On the proton-density image (SE 1500/38) at the corresponding level the invaded marrow (arrows, arrowheads) of both left arytenoid and thyroid cartilages is seen. Signal intensity is slightly increased compared with the T1 weighted image, confirming cartilage invasion. (c) Axial T1 weighted image (SE 400/38) at the glottic cord level shows invasion of the left part (arrows) of the cricoid cartilage and in the area of the anterior commissure (arrowheads). (d) Proton-density image (SE 1500/38) at the corresponding level demonstrates invaded marrow (arrows, arrowheads) of the cricoid and thyroid cartilages with slightly increased signal intensity compared with the T1 weighted image.

was invaded by laryngeal cancer in 13 of 16 patients (all men). In the remaining group of three patients, non-ossified cartilage was involved (all women).

Laryngeal cancer recurred in 10 of the 16 patients with cartilage invasion. Tumor recurrence was found in 10 of 15 patients with invaded thyroid cartilage, in three of five patients with invaded cricoid cartilage and four of six patients with invaded arytenoid cartilage. Only two of 19 patients without cartilage invasion had recurrent cancer. Laryngeal cancer recurred in four of six patients with invasion of more than one cartilage. Nine of 13 patients with invaded ossified cartilage and one of three patients with invaded nonossified cartilage had recurrent tumor.

Nine patients suffered from severe complications of radiation treatment, which required supportive measures. In four patients, including one patient who had radionecrosis, complications were followed by recurrent cancer. MR imaging did not show cartilage invasion in all five remaining patients who were suffering from severe edema or mucositis.

MR examination showed cartilage invasion in the area of the anterior commissure in one of eight patients with T1a glottic lesions (patient 17). Tumor recurred in none of these patients (Table 2). In three of four patients with a glottic lesion staged as T1b, MR imaging demonstrated cartilage invasion in the area of the anterior commissure. Two of these three patients had recurrent tumor (Table 2). Cartilage invasion was found in six of the twelve patients with a glottic lesion staged as T2. In four of these six, cancer had recurred. However, tumor also recurred in two of the other six patients, who showed no cartilage invasion (Table 2). Of two patients with T3 glottic lesions, one had cartilage invasion and neither suffered from tumor recurrence. MR examination of both T4 glottic lesion showed cartilage invasion and tumor recurred in both patients (Table 2). In both cases of T1 and T2 supraglottic cancer, cartilage invasion was not found (Table 2). Both patients remained free of disease. MR imaging showed cartilage invasion in two of

Table 2. Presence of cartilage invasion and tumor recurrence by location and stage

Tumor Type	Invasion Yes	No
Glottic		
T1a		
Recurrence	0	0
No recurrence	1	7
T1b		
Recurrence	2	0
No recurrence	1	1
T2		
Recurrence	4	2
No recurrence	2	4
T3 and T4		
Recurrence	2	0
No recurrence	1	1
Supraglottic		
T1 and T2		
Recurrence	0	0
No recurrence	0	2
T3 and T4		
Recurrence	2	0
No recurrence	0	2

four T3 and T4 supraglottic cancer and in both patients tumor did recur (Table 2). All patients with a supraglottic tumor who were without MR evidence of invasion remained free of disease (Table 2).

4. Discussion

Our patient population mostly comprises patients with smaller laryngeal cancers, who were treated with radiation therapy. In most of these patients, CT would be expected to show cartilage invasion. The present group of patients produced a higher percentage of adequate MR examinations (90%) than our previous group of patients with surgically treated cancers (approximately 83%) [13]. Obviously, patients with smaller cancers do not suffer from dyspnea and coughing as much as patients with larger tumors. The mean follow-up time in this series is 24 months and is therefore relatively brief. It has been reported that almost all recurrences of glottic cancer occur within two years. Recurrences of supraglottic cancer can be expected within up to five years [14, 15]. Therefore, results regarding patients with glottic and supraglottic lesions should be considered as preliminary.

Laryngeal cartilages are very difficult to investigate due to their irregular pattern of ossification [8, 16–21]. The hyaline cartilages may be variably composed of calcified and non-calcified cartilage, or of bone with a marrow cavity [8, 17]. In some patients, CT may suggest invasion of cartilage. Non-calcified or poorly calcified cartilage may appear as erosion or destruction on CT scans. In ossified cartilages, tumor may grossly invade the medullary space of the laryngeal cartilages, but may not be detected with CT if the surrounding bone is still intact. In a recent publication on advanced laryngeal cancer it was stated that unrecognized cartilage invasion occurs with a frequency of 25% [22]. By contrast, MR imaging accurately shows ossification patterns and allows detection of even minor cartilage invasion [11]. We have previously studied the accuracy of CT and MRI in showing cartilage invasion in 16 patients by comparing the results with histopathological findings. The two modalities were almost equal in specificity. The sensitivity to cartilage invasion was 46% for CT and 89% for MR imaging [13]. The MR appearances in the present group of 35 non-surgically treated patients demonstrated cartilage invasion in 16 patients. Cartilage invasion was found even in small glottic lesions such as T1b (three of four cases) (Table 2) or T2 (six of 12 cases) (Table 2). Generally, supraglottic cancers are less prone to invade thyroid cartilage [23]. This is in accordance with the MRI findings of our patients with small supraglottic cancers.

Invasion is nearly always confined to the portion of the cartilage that has been ossified [19, 21, 24]. However, in our series we found the nonossified cartilage to be involved in three patients with tumors clinically staged as T2, T3 and T4. In one patient with a tumor staged as T2 (case 30), we found on the proton density image a relatively small area of increased signal intensity inside nonossified cartilage. The connective tissue planes within the larynx provide a natural pathway for invasion of the ossified cartilages at their attachment to the cartilage. The most important sites are (a) the thyroid angle at the attachment of the anterior commissure tendon, (b) the attachments of the cricothyroid membrane, (c) the anterior portion of the thyroid lamina near the origin of the thyroarytenoid muscle, and (d) the capsule of the cricoarytenoid joint [18, 24].

Glottic tumors tend to invade the thyroid cartilage at the anterior commissure [19,24]. With MR imaging it is difficult to differentiate between invasion in the area of the anterior commissure and invasion into the anterior portion of the thyroid lamina near the origin of the thyroarytenoid muscles. These areas in the anterior part of the thyroid lamina are the ones mostly involved in patients with thyroid cartilage invasion (Figs. 1–3).

Cancer that invades the paraglottic space exhibits an aggresive growth pattern, infiltrating the laryngeal framework in most cases, and emerging from the confines of the larynx by direct extension between the thyroid and cricoid cartilages at the cricothyroid membrane [25, 26]. Olofsson and van Nostrand reported that only two of 27 tumors which penetrated the cricothyroid membrane did so without invading cartilage [26]. However, MR evidence of invasion of the lower edge of the thyroid lamina was only found in one patient (patient 30). Perhaps this kind of infiltration is more likely to be found in larger tumors.

Tumors of the posterior ends of the vocal cord tend to invade the arytenoid cartilage. It is reported that whenever the arytenoid cartilage is invaded, the adjacent area of the cricoid cartilage is also invaded [24]. Detection of invasion of the arytenoid cartilage may be difficult, especially if this cartilage is nonossified. It can be assumed to be invaded if surrounded by tumor. Invasion into this area is often found on the MR images. Differentiation between invasion of the arytenoid and cricoid cartilages is difficult on transverse MR images (Figs. 1–3).

Neoplastic invasion of the yellow elastic fibrocartilage of the epiglottis is amenable to radiation therapy [3]. Invasion of this type of cartilage was not investigated in this study. Our results suggest that the MR appearance of cartilage invasion in the remaining cartilages appears to have a prognostic value regarding tumor recurrence after radiation treatment. Any degree of invasion into the thyroid cartilage by small laryngeal cancers appears to increase the subsequent risk of tumor recurrence. The increased risk of tumor recurrence of T1b glottic cancers (two out of four T1b glottic lesions) agrees with reports from the literature, in which tumor recurrence of T1b lesions varies from 30 to 85% [27–29]. One might expect a correlation between the number of invaded cartilages and the extent of cartilage invasion on the one hand and the risk of tumor recurrence on the other hand. Concerning this hypothesis, no statistically significant conclusions can be drawn from our study due to insufficient numbers of patients. This limitation also applies to a possible difference in prognosis between patients in whom nonossified or ossified cartilage was invaded. In agreement with others, we find permanent serious complications, such as radionecrosis, to be rare. MR imaging, in our study, had no predictive value with regard to complications of radiation therapy, such as radionecrosis and mucositis. One of the two glottic tumors, in which MRI did not show invasion, but tumor did recur, was a large tumor that filled over a half of the paraglottic space. This may be another prognostic criteria for tumor recurrence [9].

Radiation therapy is now the preferred therapy in T1 and T2 glottic cancers in most institutions because it enables a high percentage of the patients to be cured and to retain a practically normal voice quality [16]. In most centres T3 and T4 lesions are treated with a wide-field laryngectomy, often combined with post-operative therapy [20]. Others prefer primary radiotherapy in these advanced tumors as well, keeping surgery in reserve for recurrent disease. Our study shows that MR imaging frequently demonstrates cartilage invasion, not only in T3 and T4 lesions, but even in T1b and T2 glottic lesions. It also appears that such cartilage invasion is predictive of the success of radiation therapy. Patients with even minor cartilage invasion seem to run a high risk of recurrence after radiation therapy. Therefore, in patients with cartilage invasion seen upon MR imaging, primary surgery is to be considered, i.e. partial laryngectomy for small tumors and total laryngectomy for large tumors. In patients with a small tumor with cartilage invasion in whom partial laryngectomy is not feasible and radiation therapy is the only option, follow-up should be stringent in order to detect possible recurrences in time for effective salvage treatment.

References

1. Bryce DP. Management of laryngeal cancer. J Otolaryngol 1979;8:105–108.
2. Vermund H. Role of radiotherapy in cancer of the larynx as related to the TNM system of staging. A Review. Cancer 1970;25:485–504.
3. Lederman M. Radiotherapy of cancer of the larynx. J Laryngol Otol 1970;84;867–896.
4. Goodrich WA, Lenz M. Laryngeal chondronecrosis following roentgen therapy. Amer J Roentgen 1948;60:22–28.
5. Harwood AR, Tierie AH. Radiotherapy of early glottic cancer. Part II. Int J Radiat Oncol Biol Phys 1979;5:477–482.
6. Keene M, Harwood AR, Bryce DP, van Nostrand AWP. Histopathological study of radionecrosis in laryngeal carcinoma. Laryngoscope 1982;92:173–180.
7. Million RR. The myth regarding bone or cartilage involvement by cancer and the likelihood of cure by radiotherapy. Head & Neck 1989;11:30–40.
8. Mafee MF, Schild JA, Michael AS, Choi KH, Capek V. Cartilage involvement in laryngeal carcinoma: correlation of CT and pathologic macrosection studies. J Comput Assist Tomogr 1984;8(5):969–73.
9. Isaacs JH, Mancuso AA, Mendenhall WM, Parsons PT. Deep spread patterns in CT staging of T2 squamous cell carcinoma. Otolaryngol Head Neck Surg 1988;99:455–464.
10. Castelijns JA, Doornbos J, Verbeeten B Jr., Vielvoye GJ, Bloem JL. Magnetic resonance imaging of the normal larynx. J Comput Assist Tomogr 1985;9(5):919–925.

11. Castelijns JA, Gerritsen GJ, Kaiser MC, Valk J, Jansen W, Meyer CJLM, Snow GB. MRI of normal and cancerous laryngeal cartilages: histopathologic correlation. Laryngoscope 1987;97:1085–1093.
12. Castelijns JA, Kaiser MC, Valk J, Gerritsen GJ, van Hattum AH, Snow GB. MRI of laryngeal cancer. J Comput Assist Tomogr 1987;11(1):134–140.
13. Castelijns JA, Gerritsen GJ, Kaiser MC, et al. Diagnosis of laryngeal cartilage invasion by cancer: comparison of CT and MRI. Radiology 1988;167:199–206.
14. Kirchner JA, Owen JR. Five hundred cancers of the larynx and pyriform sinus. Results of treatment by radiation and surgery. Largyngoscope 1977;81:1288–1303.
15. Fletcher GH et al. Reasons for irradiation failure in squamous cell cancer of the larynx. The Laryngoscope 1975;85:987–1003.
16. Gerritsen GJ, Valk J,van Velzen DJ, Snow GB. Computed tomography: a mandatory investigational procedure for the T-staging of advanced laryngeal cancer. Clin Otolaryngol 1986;11:307–316.
17. Hoover LA, Calcaterra TC, Walter GA, Larrson SG. Preoperative CT scan evaluation for laryngeal carcinoma: correlation with pathological findings. Laryngoscope 1984;94:310–315.
18. Silverman PM, Bossen EH, Fisher SR, Boylce Cole T, Korobkin L, Halvorsen RA. Carcinoma of the larynx and hypopharynx: computed tomographic-histopathologic correlations. Radiology 1984;151:697–702.
19. Yeager VL, Lawson C, Archer CR. Ossification of the laryngeal cartilages as it relates to computed tomography. Invest Radiol 1982;17:11–19.
20. Archer CR, Yeager VL. Computed Tomography of laryngeal cancer with histopathological correlation. Laryngoscope 1982;92:1173–1180.
21. Kirchner JA. 100 Laryngeal cancers studied by serial section. Ann Otol 1969;78:689–710.
22. Decker JW, Price JC, Godstein JC. Advanced laryngeal cancer. Relevance of pathological stage to survival and therapy. Arch Otolaryngol Head Neck Surg 1986;112:1163–1167.
23. Kirchner JA, Som ML. Clinical and histopathological observations on supraglottic cancer. Ann Otol 1971;80:638–646.
24. Yeager VL, Archer. CR, Anatomical routes of cancer invasion of laryngeal cartilages. The laryngoscope 1982;92:449.
25. Sessions DG. Surgical pathology of the larynx and hypopharynx. Laryngoscope 1975;86:814–839.
26. Olofsson J, van Nostrand AWP. Growth and spread of laryngeal carcinoma with reflections on the effect of preoperative irradiation: 139 cases studied by whole organ serial sectioning. Acta Oto-Laryngologica 1973;308:1–84.
27. Kirchner JA. Cancer at the anterior commissure of the larynx. Results with radiotherapy. Arch Otolaryngol 1970;91:524.
28. Som ML, Silver CE. The anterior commissure technique of partial laryngectomy. Arch Otolaryngol 1968;87:138–145.
29. Oloffson J, Williams GT, Ridder WD, Bryce DP. Anterior commissure carcinoma. Primary treatment with radiotherapy in 57 patients. Arch Otolaryngol 1972;95:230.

Chapter 11: General discussion

If one employs standard head and body coils, the structures of the neck are particularly difficult to image by MRI. Head coils will not cover the middle and inferior regions of the neck because the shoulders interfere with positioning. Body coils are inefficient because of the small size of the region of interest. The application of specially designed surface coils has been proved to be the ideal solution to these problems. The use of these types of coils results in a considerable improvement of the signal-to-noise ratio of the laryngeal image. It is also possible to obtain high signal resolution images with a field of view as small as possible and with a minimal slice thickness, which is necessary to demonstrate delicate laryngeal structures.

CT images are frequently degraded by streak artifacts caused by swallowing, respiratory motion and/or X-ray beam hardening. A disadvantage of MRI is that, in the present stage of the technology, examination times for MRI are considerably longer, being of the order of minutes, as against seconds for CT. Consequently, MR imaging is much more susceptible to degradation by gross motion. Occasionally (in this study in 16% of the examinations), image quality may interfere with the minimum requirements for diagnostic work-up. In agreement with Stark, we find that MR images are only minimally affected by normal respiratory movements [1]. Patients with great difficulty in swallowing, excessive coughing or patients with chronic respiratory disease and/or forced breathing are unsuitable candidates. Furthermore, due to the long examination times it is not yet possible to image laryngeal structures without motion artifacts, while performing phonation or other physiological manoeuvers. However, the recent introduction of the fast scanning technique offers new prospects [2].

Applying the MR inversion recovery technique, we could not differentiate between muscular, bony and cartilagineous structures. MR spin echo (SE) images display greater soft tissue detail. In contrast to the findings of Stark et al., images, obtained with short repetition time (TR) and short echo time (TE), are preferable for the demonstration of the laryngeal anatomy [1]. SE T1 weighted images show relevant intralaryngeal structures (intrinsic musculature and the intralaryngeal compartments), the laryngeal cartilages and extralaryngeal structures (infrahyoid muscles, vascular structures in the carotid sheath) with excellent detail and soft tissue definition. In particular, non-ossified and ossified cartilages are seen with clear contrast. Non-ossified cartilage is demonstrated with an intermediate signal intensity. Ossified cartilage has a typically three-layer appearance: high signal bone marrow being surrounded by low signal cortical rims. Cortical bone is imaged with low signal intensity due to the lack of mobile protons. Bone marrow, irrespective of the proportion of fatty and haemopoietic content, is always seen with high signal intensity. In fact, haemopoietic marrow consists of 25–50% fat.

Surgery, partial or total laryngectomy, and/or radiation therapy are the modalities of choice for the treatment of laryngeal cancer. The choice between these modalities is influenced, among other things, by the site and the extent of the lesion. In particular, the question whether cartilage invasion is present or absent is of importance. Radiation therapy, particularly at high doses, may be contra-indicated and total laryngectomy may be indicated, if cartilage invasion exists. If the cartilages are invaded by tumor, radiation often results in perichondritis, necrosis or sequestration of the cartilages, particularly if high doses of radiation are given. Furthermore, accurate assessment of the extent of the primary lesion is highly important with regards to the feasibility and the application of the various techniques of irradiation treatment.

Direct and indirect laryngoscopic examinations offer a great deal of information about the site, the volume, and the extent of the intralaryngeal lesion, but do not provide information about the submucosal extension of the lesion and some hidden regions, such as the subglottic area or areas concealed by a large tumor mass. The conventional radiological modalities, such as contrast laryngography and conventional tomography, may provide additional information about the extent of the disease. However, these modalities have been largely supplanted by CT. The introduction of CT has been a breakthrough in demonstrating the submucosal extent of the disease in the axial plane, particularly extralaryngeal spread and major cartilage invasion. CT provides helpful information about areas that may be hidden from visual inspection by bulky tumors, such as the subglottis. More importantly, it reveals submucosal extension which is not visible by other means. However, information on the extent of the tumor can only indirectly be inferred from CT images, by assessing the distortion of the laryngeal structures or narrowing of the laryngeal lumen. This study demonstrates that MR T1 weighted images appear to be more appropriate than CT in the assessment of the extent of laryngeal cancer. On T1 weighted images, tumor tissue is found with homogeneously intermediate signal intensity, slightly higher than the signal intensity of muscular tissue, but definitely lower than that of fat. Images accentuating T2 characteristics (proton density or T2 weighted images), show tumor tissue with less homogeneous signal intensity. Tumor is found with increased signal intensity, minimizing the contrast between the tumor on the one hand and muscular and cartilagineous tissues on the other. T2 weighted images have a relatively low signal-to-noise ratio. The use of proton density images is a good compromise between a reasonable signal-to-noise ratio and an adequate expression of T2 tissue characteristics.

The axial imaging technique is, above other scan directions, appropriate for the study of the site and the extent of intralaryngeal compartments (pre-epiglottic space and right and left paraglottic spaces), laryngeal cartilages as well as in extralaryngeal structures, such as the infrahyoid muscles, piriform sinus, subcutaneous fat and lymph nodes along the carotid sheath.

MRI has the advantage over CT that it is capable of imaging in the frontal and sagittal planes in a sufficiently accurate manner. On frontal images, the cranio-caudal extension of the tumor, particularly subglottic extension, and the relationship between the caudal margin of the tumor and the upper border of the cricoid, is more clearly demonstrated. The laryngeal ventricles may be seen open on frontal images, but this is not a constant finding in patients who do not have abnormalities at the level of the laryngeal ventricles. On sagittal images infiltration of the root of the tongue by tumor tissue is well visualized. The distance between the caudal margin of a supraglottic tumor and the anterior commissure can be assessed.

Three-dimensional representation of pathology, as may be demonstrated by MRI, enables calculation of the tumor volume to provide the basis for radiation therapy.

In this study we demonstrate that the main advantage of MRI over any other diagnostic modality appears to be its capability of demonstrating laryngeal cartilage invasion by cancer. This will be discussed first of all for the epiglottic cartilage.

The epiglottic cartilage consists of elastic fibrocartilage and generally does not ossify. All other laryngeal cartilages consist of hyaline cartilage and ossify at an advanced age. This study demonstrates that the vicinity of tumor to the epiglottic cartilage, as shown by MR T1 weighted, axial and sagittal images, appears to be suspicious for cartilage invasion. Using these criteria, the sensitivity of MRI in the detection of invasion of the epiglottic cartilage is much higher than that of CT. Whereas, on CT, the extent of the lesion is often underestimated due to low contrast differences between pathological tissue and pre-epiglottic fat, SE T1 weighted images show more contrast between both tissues.

The changes in hyaline cartilage are the subject of extensive discussion in the literature. In some studies it is maintained that both processes (ossification and calcification) are interrelated, whereas other authors favour the view that both processes are totally independent of each other. This confusion continues in recent reports concerning MRI of the neck area [3–5]. In this study, changes in the cartilages, as visualized by CT, are defined with the term "calcification", and changes in hyaline cartilages observed in MR images, with the corresponding term "ossification". Comparison of CT and MR images with the corresponding microscopic sections suggest that patterns of calcification and ossification agree to a certain extent.

It has been stated that CT is superior to MR imaging in depicting laryngeal cartilages and detection of cartilage invasion [6]. However, the present study demonstrates that MR imaging, by combined use of axial T1 weighted and proton density images, is more appropriate than CT for the detection of invasion of laryngeal cartilages. Due to irregular calcification and the high degree of variability of calcification between individuals, minor cartilage invasion cannot be detected by CT. Uncalcified or poorly calcified cartilage is inadequately shown by CT, and therefore erosion or destruction may thus be simulated. On the other hand, the tumor may very frequently grossly invade the medullary space of the laryngeal cartilages without destroying bony trabeculae and surrounding bone and may therefore escape detection because the presence of these bony structures allows for reconstruction of an apparently normal cartilage on CT.

Comparison of the results of CT and MRI observers indicates that MRI detects cartilage invasion with a higher accuracy and, in particular, a much higher sensitivity than does CT. Detection of invasion into hyaline cartilage (cricoid, arytenoid and thyroid cartilages) is greatly improved by the use of both T1 weighted and proton density images. T1 weighted images allow separation between pathological and normal bone marrow. Proton density images permit differentiation between non-ossified cartilage and tumor tissue.

The MR appearances in the group of 35 non-surgically treated patients demonstrated cartilage invasion in 16 patients. Cartilage invasion was found even in small glottic lesions such as T1b (three of four cases) or T2 (six of 12 cases). Generally, supraglottic cancers are less prone to invade thyroid cartilage. This is in agreement with the MRI findings of our patients with small supraglottic cancers. The most important sites are (a) the thyroid angle at the attachment of the anterior commissure tendon, (b) the anterior portion of the thyroid lamina near the origin of the thyroarytenoid muscle, and (c) the capsule of the cricoarytenoid joint. Glottic tumors tend to invade the thyroid cartilage at the anterior commissure. The area of the anterior commissure and invasion into the anterior portion of the thyroid lamina near the origin of the thyroarytenoid muscles are the ones mostly involved in patients with thyroid cartilage invasion. Tumors of the posterior ends of the vocal cord tend to invade the arytenoid cartilage. Whenever the arytenoid cartilage is invaded, the adjacent area of the cricoid cartilage is also invaded. Detection of invasion of the arytenoid cartilage may be difficult, especially if this cartilage is nonossified. It can be assumed to be invaded if surrounded by tumor. Invasion into this area is often found on the MR images. Differentiation between invasion of the arytenoid and cricoid cartilages is difficult on transverse MR images.

The MR appearance of cartilage invasion in the remaining cartilages appears to have a prognostic value regarding tumor recurrence after radiation treatment. Any degree of invasion into the thyroid cartilage by small laryngeal cancers appears to increase the subsequent risk of tumor recurrence. The increased risk of tumor recurrence of T1b glottic cancers (two out of four T1b glottic lesions) agrees with reports from the literature, in which tumor recurrence of T1b lesions varies from 30 to 85%. Patients with even minor cartilage invasion seem to run a high risk of recurrence after radiation therapy. Therefore, in patients with cartilage invasion seen upon MR imaging, primary surgery is to be considered, i.e. partial laryngectomy for small tumors and total laryngectomy for large tumors. In patients with a small tumor with cartilage invasion in whom partial laryngectomy is not feasible and radiation therapy the only option, follow-up should be stringent in order to detect possible recurrences in time for effective salvage treatment.

In this study, MRI appears to be less effective in patients suspected of having a recurrent or residual tumor after previous irradiation treatment. No distinction is possible between cancer, edema and irradiation fibrosis. This agrees with the findings of Lufkin et al. [7], but is in contrast to preliminary reports of Glazer et al. [4], in which it is maintained that MR imaging is very encouraging in evaluating the post-treatment neck.

In summary, the comparison with histological findings and statistical evaluation suggest a superiority of MR imaging over CT in delineating the site and the extent of laryngeal cancer. MRI should therefore be included in the diagnostic work-up of all patients with laryngeal cancer who have not been treated previously, with the exception of those patients with small tumors such as glottic T1 lesions. If MRI fails due to movement artifacts, claustrophobia, metallic inplants in the region of interest or if MRI is impossible in patients bearing a pacemaker or surgical clips, CT may still be necessary.

References

1. Stark DD, Moss AA, Gamsu G, Clark OH, Gooding GA, Webb WR. Magnetic resonance imaging of the neck. Part 1: normal anatomy. radiology 1984; 150: 447–454.
2. Van der Meulen P. Groen JP, Cuppen JJM. Very fast MR Imaging by filed echoes and small angle excitation. Magn Reson Imaging 1985; 3: 297–299.
3. Wortham DG, Hoover LA, Lufkin RB, Fu YS. Magnetic resonance imaging of the larynx; a correlation with histologic sections. Otolaryngol head and neck surg 1986; 94: 123–133.
4. Glazer HS, Niemeyer JH. Balfe DM et al. Neck neoplasms: MR Imaging. Part 1. Initial evaluation. Radiology 1986; 160: 343–348.
5. Lufkin RB, Hanafee WN. Application of surface coils to MR anatomy of the larynx. AJNR 1985; 6: 491–497.
6. McArdle CB, Bailley BJ, Amparo EG. Surface coil magnetic resonance imaging of the normal larynx. Arch Otolaryngol Head and Neck Surg 1986; 112: 616–622.
7. Lufkin RB, Hanafee WN, Wortham D, Hoover L. Larynx and hypopharynx: MR imaging with surface coils. Radiology 1986; 158: 747–754.

Index

SERIES IN RADIOLOGY

1. J.O. Op den Orth: *The Standard Biphasic-contrast Examination of the Stomach and Duodenum.* Method, Results, and Radiological Atlas. 1979 ISBN 90-247-2159-8
2. J.L. Sellink and R.E. Miller: *Radiology of the Small Bowel.* Modern Enteroclysis Technique and Atlas. 1982 ISBN 90-247-2460-0
3. R.E. Miller and J. Skucas: *The Radiological Examination of the Colon.* Practical Diagnosis. 1983 ISBN 90-247-2666-2
4. S. Forgács: *Bones and Joints in Diabetes Mellitus.* 1982 ISBN 90-247-2395-7
5. Gy. Németh and H. Kuttig (eds.): *Isodose Atlas for Use in Radiotherapy.* 1981 ISBN 90-247-2476-7
6. J. Chermet: *Atlas of Phlebography of the Lower Limbs.* Including the Iliac Veins. 1982 ISBN 90-247-2525-9
7. B.K. Janevski: *Angiography of the Upper Extremity.* 1982 ISBN 90-247-2684-0
8. M.A.M. Feldberg: *Computed Tomography of the Retroperitoneum.* An Anatomical and Pathological Atlas with Emphasis on the Fascial Planes. 1983 ISBN 0-89838-573-3
9. L.E.H. Lampmann, S.A. Duursma and J.H.J. Ruys: *CT Densitometry in Osteoporosis.* The Impact on Management of the Patient. 1984 ISBN 0-89838-633-0
10. J.J. Broerse and T.J. Macvittie: *Response of Different Species to Total Body Irradiation.* 1984 ISBN 0-89838-678-0
11. C. L'Herminé: *Radiology of Liver Circulation.* 1985 ISBN 0-89838-715-9
12. G. Maatman: *High-resolution Computed Tomography of the Paranasal Sinuses, Pharynx and Related Regions.* Impact of CT Identification on Diagnosis and Patient Management. 1986 ISBN 0-89838-802-3
13. C. Plets, A.L. Baert, G.L. Nijs and G. Wilms: *Computer Tomographic Imaging and Anatomic Correlation of the Human Brain.* A Comparative Atlas of Thin CT-scan Sections and Correlated Neuro-anatomic Preparations. 1987 ISBN 0-89838-811-2
14. J. Valk: *MRI of the Brain, Head, Neck and Spine.* A Teaching Atlas of Clinical Applications. 1987 ISBN 0-89838-957-7
15. J.L. Sellink: *X-Ray Differential Diagnosis in Small Bowel Disease.* A Practical Approach. 1988 ISBN 0-89838-351-X
16. Th.H.M. Falke (ed.): *Essentials of Clinical MRI.* 1988 ISBN 0-89838-353-6
17. B.D. Fornage: *Endosonography.* 1989 ISBN 0-7923-0047-5
18. R. Chisin (ed.): *MRI/CT and Pathology in Head and Neck Tumors.* A Correlative Study. 1989 ISBN 0-7923-0227-3
19. G. Gozzetti, A. Mazziotti, L. Bolondi and L. Barbara (eds.): *Intraoperative Ultrasonography in Hepato-biliary and Pancreatic Surgery.* A Practical Guide. With Contributions by Y. Chapuis, J.-F. Gigot and P.-J. Kestens. 1989 ISBN 0-7923-0261-3
20. A.M.A. De Schepper and H.R.M. Degryse: *Magnetic Resonance Imaging of Bone and Soft Tissue Tumors and Their Mimics.* A Clinical Atlas. With Contributions by F. De Belder, L. van den Houwe, F. Ramon, P. Parizel and N. Buyssens. 1989 ISBN 0-7923-0343-1
21. J.O. Barentsz, F.M.J. Debruyne and S.H.J. Ruijs: *Magnetic Resonance Imaging of Carcinoma of the Urinary Bladder.* With a Forword by H. Hricak and R. Hohenfellner. 1990 ISBN 0-7923-0838-7
22. C. Depré, J.A. Melin, W. Wijns, R. Demeure, F. Hammer and J. Pringot: *Atlas of Cardiac MR Imaging with Anatomical Correlations.* Foreword by Alexander R. Margulis. 1991 ISBN 0-7923-0941-3

MIX
Papier aus verantwortungsvollen Quellen
Paper from responsible sources
FSC® C105338

If you have any concerns about our products,
you can contact us on
ProductSafety@springernature.com

In case Publisher is established outside the EU,
the EU authorized representative is:
Springer Nature Customer Service Center GmbH
Europaplatz 3, 69115 Heidelberg, Germany

Printed by Libri Plureos GmbH
in Hamburg, Germany